TENACITY

A Physician's Struggle with Parkinson's Disease

JONATHAN LESSIN, MD

NEWMAN SPRINGS PUBLISHING
320 Broad Street
Red Bank, NJ 07701

First originally published by Newman Springs Publishing 2018

This memoir depicts many medical concepts and procedures from
Dr. Jonathan Lessin's life. Although he is a physician, he is not
trained in neurology, neurosurgery, or physical therapy. This memoir
is not intended to offer, or to be used as a substitute for, the medical
advice of physicians or health care providers. The reader should
consult a physician/health care provider in all matters relating to his
or her health. The author and publisher do not assume and hereby
disclaim any liability for any loss, damage or suffering to any person
reading or following the information in this book.

ISBN 978-1-64096-107-4 (Paperback)
ISBN 978-1-64096-108-1 (Digital)

Printed in the United States of America

I too live with Parkinson's, and I feel so fortunate to have had physical therapy with Lisa Ebb. She got me moving again through the *big* physical therapy regimen, and mentioned Dr. Lessin's rock climbing support group. Rock climbing has become a passion, and even better, I have become friends with Dr. Lessin.

Anyone with Parkinson's disease can fight back. Jonathan Lessin's story shows dramatically that although Parkinson's can devastate a career (Parkinson's ended my career as surely as Dr. Lessin's) and can devastate one's confidence and self-worth (imagine 'freezing' in a doorway, and holding up a crowd of people for minutes), a Parkie can fight back with appropriate medicine, DBS surgery when efficacious, knowledge, and a supportive family.

The fight, though, begins in one's own inner core. We have to fight tenaciously every day, every hour, every minute. Jonathan Lessin's memoir *Tenacity* is an inspiring account of this fight—a lesson and guide to review over and over.

—Michael Mastromichalis

As a fellow Parkie with DBS, there is much that I was able to relate to in his memoir. I especially enjoyed how he intertwined his expedition in the Canadian subarctic as a teen, and how those experiences helped solidify his character throughout his adult life in the way he coped with challenges, decision making, and leadership.

On a personal note, Jon has had a profound positive impact on my quality of life through his guidance on DBS issues. He has also encouraged me to participate in the ski program at BOEC. I look forward to spending time with him and fellow Parkies.

—Robert B. Ettleman, DDS, MAGD, CEO,
Gulf Coast Dental Outreach

This memoir is dedicated to my wife, Cheryl, and my daughters, Julie and Brittany, who are all beautiful inside and out. Your enduring love and support allow me to continue to live a fulfilling life.

I love you always.

FOREWORD

Tenacity is a story about courage and hope. Merriam-Webster defines the word *tenacious* as an adjective meaning "not easily stopped or pulled apart," "firm and strong," and "persistent in maintaining, adhering to or seeking something desired or valued." Jonathan Lessin's story fully embodies the term *tenacious* and all it implies.

When faced with the diagnosis of Parkinson's disease, Jon chose to arm himself with knowledge and support. He pushed himself to learn and achieve in all areas of his life. Despite "freezing attacks" and a growing dependence on his medication to feel balanced, Jon sought ways to cope, and ways to overcome the growing challenges of his condition.

Never once did he imagine giving up on his dreams. Astonishingly, Jon didn't cut back on his life's wish list—he added to it. Jonathan Lessin is a man of courage, and a man of hope. His refusal to see himself as a passenger, and his desire to be the driver behind the handlebars, serves as heart-pounding and blood-pulsing inspiration to all who find themselves faced with adversity.

It is my hope that each person who comes upon this book will feel moved and encouraged to seek out the most in life. As Jon says, "Life is not a sprint; enjoy the ride."

—Hillary Dodge, editor, Hidden Thoughts Press

ACKNOWLEDGMENTS

Thank you to Raj whose never failing optimism
inspired me to write my memoir.

INTRODUCTION

I wasn't born with tenacity. I wasn't born with self-confidence or perseverance. I wasn't born with bravery or the willingness to go for it and take risks. What follows is a memoir, which chronicles the life events that taught me persistence, resolve, and gave me the necessary courage to take the risks required to have a fulfilling life in the face of the challenges I would encounter later in life.

After several years of training, and nineteen years of working as a cardiac anesthesiologist in my dream job, I was confronted with the debilitating effects of Young Onset Parkinson's disease. I held on and continued to work and teach residents for six years after my diagnosis. Finally, I decided to take myself out of the game before I ever had a complaint from a patient or surgeon. In my early retirement, I have used my learned tenacity and persistence to fight the effects of this progressive movement disorder.

Tenacity covers several events from my early life that strengthened me. Although I had two amazing sisters, I never had any brothers to challenge me. My best friend, Willie, fulfilled this role. He and I met in the seventh grade. He encouraged me to fight back against some bullies and showed me that most bullies are actually cowards. He also taught me the value of physical strength and endurance as we learned to lift weights and run together. Willie and I would play fight all the time, which built my confidence, but most importantly, we developed the use of humor to help us face challenges. This lessened the pain and allowed us to persevere.

Willie came to visit me, while I was recovering from my Deep Brain Stimulator implantation, to make me laugh. The first few weeks following the procedure can be challenging because of brain swelling. Also, the DBS hadn't yet been activated. Willie knocked on the door, and it took me a good ten minutes to get off the couch and shuffle to the front door.

Willie's first words to me were, "You had better call your neurosurgeon, this s—t ain't workin'!"

I stood, frozen in laughter for ten minutes. I knew my best friend was there.

We all learn different methods to overcome adversity. Human nature is resilient. No matter what cards we are dealt, we will somehow persist and proceed. Guided by our values, the experiences we have in life shape the way we use our own personal strengths in the face of challenge. I hope this book inspires anyone faced with a life-changing illness to look inward and find the strength to continue toward their values in their own way.

PERSEVERANCE—PART 1

Per·se·ver·ance—continued effort to do or achieve
something despite difficulties, failure, or opposition.
—Merriam-Webster Dictionary

The day's temperature had peaked at eighty degrees Fahrenheit, and even though it was summer, during the two-hour nights, it dipped down into the thirties. We were close to the permafrost of the Arctic tundra. The air temperature mimicked the dead of winter while we slept, so we had to cocoon ourselves in down sleeping bags. With the mornings awakenings, we were greeted by our frozen socks and boots to remind us that, although it was late summer, we were far from home.

This was polar bear country. However, the fiercest animals that we contended with daily were the mosquito and her best friend, the black fly. Every night, once the sun disappeared from the sky, the gloaming light would remain for hours due to our proximity to the North Pole at that time of year. The flying terrorists would sense their warm targets, and their low-pitched humming would be a three-minute warning for us to dive into our tents before we were attacked by hundreds of these biting insects. The night consisted of mostly a semidark, dusk-like light with about two hours of real darkness in the middle of our sleep. The technicolor Northern Lights were visible almost every night, but we would have had to wake during that short period of darkness if we wanted a glimpse of them.

I was sixteen. I was experiencing the most challenging time of my life or so I thought. This excursion was my first time in the Arctic, as it was for Pitt, Watt, and Fred; but Rory, our twenty-year-old trip leader, had been there several times prior. I first met Rory at Camp Manitowish in northern Wisconsin two summers earlier. He was my counselor and would lead weeklong canoe trips in the nearby lakes. Rory was a giant in my eyes. He appeared fearless, invincible, experienced, and knowledgeable. He had faith in me, because we had been on shorter canoe trips in Wisconsin and southern Canada in previous summers. Rory chose me as one of his campers to experience this ultimate excursion with him. I would later realize that his trust in me was the beginning of my own journey to confidence and strength.

This wilderness trip covered six hundred sixty miles in five weeks through Northern Saskatchewan and Manitoba, which is about an inch and a half on most globes. At one point on the trip, we would be within four hundred miles of the Arctic Circle.

I never thought of myself as strong before this excursion. I had a history of losing fights in junior high school, and endured the teasing that a black eye brought as a result. I had this inherent sense of defeatism. I excelled in math and science, but that wasn't the currency of success in my school. As a child, my school was my universe. I went to the first day of football practice in high school, just to be sent home by the coach to avoid injury.

"But my dad said I could play safety," I begged.

"Son, the safest thing for you to do would be to go home," replied the coach.

I guess I needed to be challenged in a new way to find out how strong I could be. A new confidence in my mental and physical abilities was waiting to be born in that frozen ground during the summer of 1980. This wilderness trip would prove to be an extremely memorable and confidence-building experience.

We were just five kids out in the true wilderness, miles away from the comfort and safety of society. For the duration, we didn't see another human being, a car, a phone, or even an electrical outlet.

Looming in our minds was the constant smoldering anxiety that we had to rely on our training and, moreover, each other for our safety, navigation, nutrition, and shelter. There was no Plan B.

Our only vehicles for the trip were two fiberglass canoes, which naturally became a burden to carry when trekking off the water. One was yellow, the other green. The first was known as Banana Boat. The second we affectionately named Collard Green. Rory would always paddle in the stern of Banana Boat. He would handpick his bowman daily, and it was such an honor to be chosen. Unwittingly, our team of five would learn a lot about ourselves that summer. Back then, we didn't know that the small challenges created by our trek across northern Canada would give us skills we would use for the rest of our lives.

The first two hundred miles of our course consisted of a chain of calm water lakes created by ancient glaciers. Beginning in Wollaston Lake, we followed a chain of lakes known as the Cochrane River lake chain. We were in true wilderness as gorgeous as it was dangerous. Our biggest fear during the trip was an encounter with the largest predator to humans, the polar bear. One of the ways we dealt with the constant threat was to empower ourselves with enough knowledge that we could differentiate between reality and myth and also have a concrete plan as to what to do during an encounter.

Polar bears will eat humans. They can stand up to twelve feet tall and extend their necks and, by pure size, intimidate their prey. We had practiced a plan to stand together and yell in a way to look larger to the bear than we were individually. In this way, one times five equals twenty. This trick has been known to work, but luckily, we never had to use it.

The lay of the land had been created by advancing and retreating ice over millions of years. Rivers continued flowing under the icebergs. The sand carried by those currents would eventually clog those tunnels beneath the icebergs. What remained after the ice receded was beautiful tube formations, which made a spectacular beach for lunches and swimming during the brief period midday when it would reach eighty degrees.

The small creeks that connected the lakes were not always passable in our canoes, so we had to carry them for the short walk between one and the next. This flat water part of the trip only covered fifteen miles each day, but it required twice as much paddling effort than the forty-five miles we covered later on the faster flowing North Seal River. These two sections of the trip were separated by seventeen miles of a dryland watershed. We had to carry all of our belongings on our backs and shoulders along moose trails and creek beds during the dry sections of our journey, an act called portaging.

The portages can be very challenging, and the shoulder pain created by packs and the canoes was exquisite—so much so that we would stop often during these treks. It was important to find a stump or rock to place our packs on so that it was possible to get going again without help hoisting them back up. Similarly, for a canoe carrier, it was crucial to find a bridge tree, which looked like big V, in which to wedge the canoe to allow us to rest, then begin again with little effort.

The defining test of my tenacity took place during a relatively long watershed portage. The air was misty and cold, and there was a powerful silence where the sounds of the dried-up creek used to roar. I felt an intense awareness of how alone we really were—hundreds of miles away from the comfort and support of society. We had five packs, and three of them were very heavy, weighing over fifty pounds, and containing the next four weeks' worth of freeze-dried breakfasts, lunches, and dinners.

Getting each pack mounted on ones back was a two-man effort. Walking with the pack was not only taxing, but also awkward. It required a bent-over posture to both support the weight and to relieve the intense shoulder pain. We would be jolted backward off our feet if we stood straight up. The canoes were heavier, but easier to mount and carry, so two of us had to double up with a pack and a canoe. I didn't think of myself as the biggest or strongest of the four of us, but Rory could see that I was up for the challenge. The skinny little guy who was sent home by the football coach was now going to prove to himself that he could do it.

The first day of this watershed crossing was life-changing. I was terrified. The fear probably stemmed from being so separated from society's safety net. I was going to be last to go with a heavy burden to carry, and there was no defined trail. After paddling lakes all morning, we had come to the highly anticipated seventeen-mile watershed crossing on dry land. It began in a dried-up creek bed with a moose trail running alongside. I hoped the moose knew where they were going. I hoped the moose weren't around.

Trekking on slippery, moss-covered rock in the cold mist, we proceeded with our usual routine. I helped the other four mount up with their food and utility packs first. Rory carried the other canoe, which he flipped onto his shoulders. When they were all loaded up, they promptly took off before I could join them. I had one lightweight soft pack full of clothes and sleeping bags and one canoe. I was sixteen years old, and I was alone. My job was to load myself up with a pack on my back and a canoe on my shoulders, climb out of the creek bed up the muddy bank onto the moose trail, and catch up to my friends without getting injured or lost.

I had practiced hoisting a canoe before, but that was on level ground without a pack on my back. As the eighty-pound canoe landed on my shoulders, I had to be directly underneath it with a firm foothold and center of gravity going straight through me. If unbalanced, the extremely top-heavy conglomeration of me, the pack, and the canoe would fall onto the rocks, injuring the canoe or more impact-fully me. Rory trusted me. And so did I.

I reached deep down inside to find the bravery and resolve I needed to continue the journey. I forced myself to ignore fear and the concern that there was no Plan B. I just had to envision success.

The rocks were slippery, so I slipped the pack on before hoisting the canoe and climbing up the muddy creek bank. I became my own cheerleader.

"Come on, Jon, you can do this!" I said aloud. "One, two, three..."

And with that, Collard Green was securely mounted on my shoulders, and I was out of the creek bed. I needed to find the moose trail and keep moving. Under the canoe, my feeling of pride and accomplishment was growing. My eyes were full of sweat, and the mosquitoes and black flies were swarming under the canoe and feasting on my arms. I had to ignore the stinging bites of the mosquitoes as well as the painful, bleeding bites of the black flies. The sweat dripping into the fresh bites added a burning sensation. I had to be careful not to give in to the temptation of swatting at them. Keeping my hands on the boat was of utmost importance.

Assuring myself that the bow of the canoe was down, I followed the trail and used the canoe to move the brush out of the way. I had never walked more than a quarter mile carrying a canoe, but somehow I found myself two miles into the portage and encountered an unexpected reward in the middle. I was so relieved to hear my friends joyously splashing around in water. This was supposed to be a dry watershed crossing for two days. A small and beautiful lake was a nice surprise halfway through—an oasis. I walked right into it, flipped the canoe into the water, and plopped the personal pack on the shore. I was elated to enter the lake and let the cool water wash over my painful bug bites. I rejoiced in that small victory of the day.

Being isolated in the Arctic tundra taught me how to go for it, never to tire nor give up. A person never knows how close he or she is to success. Although life is essentially a team sport, sometimes you don't have a team. You need to dig deep and find the team within yourself. It's the team of courage, planning, intelligence, humor, and self-esteem that I used because I had nobody else.

Usually, we fed off each other's help. One could argue that this is what makes one plus one equal three. With the journey into the Arctic tundra, we formed such a group. The pack carriers couldn't have started their journey alone, because hoisting the pack is a two-man job. I had to start alone; there was no choice. For me, one had to equal three. Even though that experience taught me the value of willpower, I think, more importantly, I learned the value of not being alone in the first place.

At the time, I had no way to know how incredibly valuable the celebration of small victories would become as I battled Parkinson's disease more than a quarter of a century later. In reality, most strength and courage is not found in our muscles. We don't have to train for it, and it doesn't always require special skill and coordination. Persistence and tenacity are of the highest importance, and we can usually accomplish much more as a team than as the sum of its individuals.

WEATHERING THE STORM

That which does not kill us makes us stronger.
—Friedrich Nietzsche

As a child and teen, I spent most of my summers at camp. My final experience was the summer following my freshman year in college. It was my second year as a sailing counselor at Camp Seagull in North Carolina, which is a big sailing camp at the mouth of the Neuse River just where it meets the Pamlico Sound. The river there is five miles across and fewer than two miles from the sound that is as unprotected as open ocean. The water was always cool and brackish. By mid-July, it was teeming with jellyfish. There were even a couple of small sharks whose fins we'd see rarely, but which emerged enough for us to notice and remain wary of them. However, the most dangerous element in that water wasn't the stinging or biting animals. I told my campers, "The jellies won't kill you, and the sharks are more afraid of you than you are of them."

No, the scariest things on the river were the storms that would arise out of nowhere. Once or twice a summer, we would see storms complete with high winds, copious lightning, and enormous waves that could toss a person around like a ragdoll.

That summer, I became the Sunfish fleet captain. I obtained this post by working as hard as I possibly could during the two-week presession getting camp ready. I was hoping to get noticed by the sailing director for this promotion, and it worked. The high post of captaincy gave me the responsibility of maintaining the integrity of a fleet of fifty Sunfish, as well as the safety of all campers sailing them. These are small boats with a single sail, easily handled by one or two people. Of course, I didn't do this job alone; I had other counselors under my direction. Still, I felt and held the ultimate responsibility for my campers.

One morning that summer, my concerns were redirected to worrying for my own life as a result of a sneak attack—the perfect storm.

The entire Sunfish fleet was on the river. All boats were sailing that morning, which meant between fifty and a hundred campers were out on the water, when the emergency siren sounded announcing the storm. We had fifty Sunfish, eight Lightnings, six Lasers, and over one hundred fifty campers out on the water. I was an eighteen-year-old fleet captain, solo in a baby whaler with only a 9.9-horsepower outboard motor and a tiller throttle. My goal was to go as quickly as possible to direct the boats in and have all campers return safely to shelter. I also needed to secure the Sunfish fleet, but that wasn't worth risking my own life.

Although I couldn't see the dark, angry clouds that others saw from the observation tower, I knew a fierce summer squall was on its way. The calm before the storm was the giveaway; it was dead. All that I could hear was the high-pitched humming coming from the motors of our boats gearing up for rescue, and the crackle of sails flopping back and forth in no wind. The horizon looked as if God had swiped a coat of dark gray paint across it, and it began to get dark. The birds had left the sky. Even the bugs were gone. I could smell the electrical tension in the air as if the clouds were trying to hold back the first bolt of lightning. As I towed multiple sailboats in, sometimes two at a time, the wind began to pick up. The mouth of the Neuse was morphing from an eerily calm span of water to a gusty washing machine with multidirectional currents.

Although the whitecaps were intimidating, I was able to bring in all of the campers on Sunfish boats. Then I began to head out to the Lightnings to transport as many campers as I could to safety. Lightnings are larger sailboats, which are a bit more seaworthy than Sunfish or even the small motorboat that I was in. They hold as many as eight people, and a lightning strike to the mast would most likely go straight to the water, leaving the occupants untouched. Most of these boats were stranded out in the middle of the river and had thrown out a sea anchor (which was an anchor off the bow attached to a life jacket) just to keep the bow into the wind. Each time I pulled up, I would leave a counselor on the boat. The younger campers were more than willing to abandon their counselors to come with me in hopes of making it to shore.

After a few roundtrips, I became completely disoriented. The wind had strengthened, and the waters began to churn. Visibility was lost, and lightning began to strike hard around my boat. It seemed as though a higher power had opened the gates of hell, and I was getting dangerously close to purgatory. In that moment, I was sure that God was calling all the shots, and I began to pray.

I managed to throw out a sea anchor, and take cover under a spinnaker sail that I had in the boat, all while begging God to let me live. Harsh rain pelted the sail. The electrical lightning strikes were becoming more frequent, rapidly approaching my boat.

This may or may not have qualified as a near-death experience, but I felt sure it did. On that day, I became very close to God. With the crashing waves, I felt as if I could speak directly to him.

As I implored him to spare my life, I frantically strategized to maximize my chances of survival. I first tried to don my lifejacket. I should have been wearing it in the first place, because then I would have realized it was way too small. I tried to stay calm as I reminded myself that I knew exactly what to do in a terrifying situation like this one. I had gone to camp for years, and procedure in a squall had been repeatedly drilled into all of our heads.

I tied the anchor to the bow and put the lifejacket on it. Tossing it in the water would keep the bow into the wind and thus keep the water out of the boat. This would minimize the chance of flipping over. All I had left was the spinnaker. Although it offered little protection, it kept some of the rain off me. I made it into a spray skirt by tying it to the gunwales in order to keep the boat and myself dry. Finding the horn, I was able to blast SOS (three short, three long, three short) in case someone was looking for me.

I knew the maneuvers; I had taught them to campers over and over. Procedure in a squall: I'm going to add Pray to God to that list.

Although I tried to remain calm as I performed the entire checklist, it just wasn't enough. This was a storm coming from a power much greater than me. I needed his help.

I lay shivering, wet and cold, under that sail for a long time. Lighting would strike every few minutes, and I would thank God each time for sparing me. I didn't know it, but I was staying with the storm and drifting rapidly toward the ocean. The waves were slapping me in the face, and the thunder and lightning kept scolding me angrily, while at the same time letting me live.

It seemed like an eternity, but probably only thirty minutes had passed since the storm rolled in; my bosses took personnel inventory and noticed I was missing. Thank God (literally) that my bosses used the same emergency protocol that kept campers and staff safe since the camp's creation. By that point, the storm passed the camp and was heading out to sea with me still aboard, praying to God to keep me alive and safe.

Despite my terror and the harsh weather conditions, I had a moment of clarity. Inexplicably, I had a strong feeling that I was going to be okay. I became very calm, and my mind became clear. I didn't know how, but I knew the rescue boat was on the way. I sensed something telling me to look up over the boat's gunwale. I crawled out from beneath the spinnaker sail and made my way to the edge where I saw my rescue boat—the big inboard tender—heading in my direction from the horizon. I hadn't yet realized that I was two miles away from camp and drifting toward Pamlico Sound.

As my rescuers from camp approached my boat, I panicked and jumped into the water to swim toward them. Climbing the ladder into the rescue boat, I immediately apologized for leaving the boat behind. However, as the apology left my mouth, I suddenly realized that a human life was much more important than any material thing, no matter the monetary value.

When we finally arrived back at camp, I was surprised to see that life had gone on as usual without me. Everyone was already at lunch, like the storm was just a story and not an actual terror. Not everyone had downplayed the storm that just passed, however. The camp director publicly thanked me for my service that morning, but all I could think about was how scared I had been. I walked into the mess hall after my adventure, soaking wet and knees still shaking; but I also had a sense of resolve, accomplishment, and a greater faith in myself.

From that day, I would take with me the value of staying calm in the face of fear, using the knowledge I had at my disposal, and taking action whenever I could to do exactly what I knew I needed to do.

WHO AM I?

Be yourself; everyone else is already taken.
—Oscar Wilde

My family story began in early twentieth-century America when my grandparents—who at that time were two young boys, a baby girl, and a toddler, emigrated in steerage from Ukraine and Belarus through Ellis Island. Like many Jewish refugees, they were escaping pogroms and Russian oppression.

My father's father, Maurice Lessin, born in Vitebsk, Belarus—the youngest and only boy among six siblings—arrived in America at age ten in 1905 with ten rubles in his pocket and an identity tag on his lapel. His father, a forester, had died in a logging accident when Maurice was two years old. Passage was paid by a cousin in Brooklyn in exchange for work in the family dry goods store where Maurice lived in the basement.

Mischa Lustok, my mom's dad, came over in a similar way fifteen years later. He ended up in Milwaukee with his parents and made his way through college and eventually medical school. There he started the family business—medicine. As a cardiologist, he would be the first of fifteen doctors in our family. Eventually, I would be the twelfth.

My parents were amazing role models to my two sisters and me. Both of my sisters are very giving people and work with people with disabilities. Jenni, my elder sister, helped autistic children and their families as a behavioral pediatrician. Tina, five years younger than I am, has helped counsel those who are physically and mentally challenged to help them work and, most recently, was a sign language interpreter. My father, the third doctor in the family, is a very accomplished hematologist/oncologist. He climbed the academic ladder quickly and became a full professor of medicine in his early thirties.

What is interesting is that I didn't inherit his love of academic medicine. Although my father became an internationally recognized physician, he rarely brought his work home with him. I believe it was his humbleness and modesty that had the greatest impact on me.

In my mother's eyes, I could do no wrong. She taught me compassion and empathy. She had a way of redirecting me as a child without raising her voice, which I brought with me as I became an instructor to anesthesiology residents. Being the first boy after a long line of girls in the Lustok family gave me special status. According to Mom, I was fantastic at everything I tried, which did wonders for my self-confidence.

The truth is I wasn't so good at everything. It is said that Parkinson's disease begins at birth and in retrospect, there were many signs early on. Although I was naturally comfortable with balancing sports, such as snow and waterskiing, windsurfing, and bicycling, I was frustrated by the activities that required aiming a ball. I couldn't understand why I was horrible at shooting a basketball or why, as a catcher, I would continuously throw the baseball back over the pitcher's head. Why was it so easy for my friends? Why did I love to play the drums, but really have trouble keeping the beat?

*****

My earliest memory was when I was two. My father took the family to Paris for a year so he could study leukemia with a famous hematologist there. We were traveling by ship, and I can still visualize the wooden planks onto the ship and how high above the water they were. The ship was full of kids. My memories of that voyage center around the fear induced by the other children who kept turning out the lights in the playroom, because they knew I would be afraid of the dark. My guardian angel on that ship was my sister, Jenni, who protected me and yelled at the other children to leave me alone.

We lived in Paris for a year. I was so proud every day to be assigned the task of carrying home fresh baguettes from the market.

Little things like this add to a person's own self-worth and ripple into the rest of life.

By the time I was in medical school, I had enough self-confidence to convince Cheryl to date and later marry me. The twelve-year-old Jon could never have done this. My marriage to Cheryl, and my two beautiful daughters, Julie and Brittany, has added immeasurable value to my journey.

*****

One of the days I will always remember was the day I met the girl of my dreams. She was the girl with whom I would spend the rest of my life.

I was at the annual University of Maryland Medical School retreat, normally held for first year medical students. I went as a second-year student to meet girls.

She walked into the dining room at the Deep Creek Lake resort, and I was struck down by her smile as if I had been hit by lightning. She had asymmetrical hair, because she had recently returned from Europe, and that was the new style… I guess. She was gorgeous. I knew I had to meet her. A mutual friend told me that she would join us waterskiing that day on a boat that I had arranged.

I took a deep breath, gathered my courage, and walked up to her. "I hear you want to waterski today."

She replied, "I am already going with a guy named Jon. Oh, and by the way, our boat is full."

She thought she had gotten rid of me. What she didn't know was that I was Jon. As we spent the day together with mutual friends, I became more and more attracted to her. I just had to go out with her. All she could talk about was that she wanted to marry a surgeon. Over the next year, we became friends, and as I made it my goal to become her boyfriend, she was trying as hard as she could to get me a date with somebody else! I was an expert at being shot down by her.

Once I got the nerve to approach her, I said, "I heard there is a great movie out this weekend."

She sarcastically replied, "Okay, well, you have fun with that!"

I even got tickets to an Eddie Murphy concert that she said she would go to, but when I showed up to pick her up, her sister was there to go with me! Can't a man take a hint?

I finally had given up when I got a call that she owed me dinner, because I had helped her with a class. Tony Cheng's, the best Chinese restaurant in Baltimore, would be our first date in my mind, if not hers.

That night inadvertently must have hooked her. It had snowed almost a foot, and she was shocked when I showed up anyway. She watched me put chains on my car. I spent the dinner telling her about my 660-mile wilderness trip across the Arctic tundra. Hadn't everyone done that? I still didn't think I had a chance at the boyfriend thing, so I didn't even try to kiss her.

That was another accidental point in my favor. A few weeks later, I gave her a ride home from a "happy hour," and as I dropped her off, she kissed me! Wow! Out of the friend zone! Pretty soon, we were together on stage dancing with George Winston!

We dated for six years before the best wedding ever seen on the face of the Earth. During that time, I fell completely in love with her. It wasn't because she was so beautiful that my mother said, "She is so pretty, I can't look away." It wasn't because of how uncontrollably happy I felt every time I saw her or how she lit up a room with her smile when she walked in. The moment that clinched it for me was when I was sick with strep throat and she put me in her bed and cared for me for four days. The kindness in her heart showed what love really is.

We had the best wedding known to man in May 1993. As a combined Jewish, Catholic, and Filipino wedding, it was huge, and everyone had a great time. We squeezed 325 guests into a chapel meant to fit only 275, all there to see my beautiful bride. Eventually, she would become an internationally known surgeon.

If I was asked how I knew I wanted to marry Cheryl, I'd have to say I just knew. I was sure that my life wouldn't have been as great without her. I didn't know then how important her loving support would be.

POKIN'

What would you do if you weren't afraid?
—Spencer Johnson

On my father's workbench sat a vise used to hold things to be worked on. For some unknown reason, I and my best friend Willie would put our hands in the vise at the same time and crank it tighter and tighter until one of us couldn't take the pain anymore and screamed for mercy. As a couple of junior high schoolers, this was the nature of our relationship. Willie seemed to want me to test my pain tolerance at all times to get the most out of life. He would always talk to me as if he were pokin' me in the chest to get his point across. I would receive letters from Willie in college, and he would actually insert the word *pokin'* in parentheses at the end as if it were the only way I would listen. He was my best friend.

I first met Willie on a religious school retreat during the first year of Cabin John junior high school. He had thick, black, curly hair, which he parted in the middle, "cool" back then. He had forgotten a hairbrush and asked to borrow mine. I reluctantly said yes, and watched him hang upside down on his bed and bury that brush into his thick hair. I never used it again.

While I slept on this weekend retreat, some of the other kids thought it would be funny to put shaving cream on my face so that I would eventually wake up in the middle of the night, rub it into my eyes, then feel as if they were on fire. My new friend, Willie, was not involved. I was intrigued as to why these bullies targeted me and not him. Willie did the best thing for me that a friend could do. He didn't fight my battles for me. He knew that most bullies were actu-

28

ally cowards and picked on those who wouldn't fight back. Willie encouraged me to retaliate. It only required one fight to change my reputation and get the bullies off my back.

I couldn't wait until one of those kids gave me a reason to attack. I had been afraid my whole life up to that point. I had pent-up anger, which stemmed from elementary school bus stop encounters with bullies. These guys actually had very low self-esteem, and made themselves feel stronger by attacking those who seemed weaker. I wasn't physically weaker at that time, but I had low confidence in my abilities. I was afraid.

Willie changed all of that. He was simply on my side. I had enough. The first derogatory comment I heard that morning set me off. I attacked. I attacked with the power of years of aggravation from my own fear. I attacked this poor kid, and kept fighting until the teachers separated us. Then I attacked some more. It wasn't that I knew that Willie would jump in and rescue me if I needed it. It wasn't that I knew the teachers would break it up. I was just tired of the fear, and had to prove to myself that I could do it. I needed to feed my own self-confidence.

Nobody bothered me again. Until...I encountered the same type of bullying as an adult. This time, I dealt with it right off the bat. At my third job as an anesthesiologist, I was working in a private practice doing anesthesia for all types of cases as well as heart surgery. I had worked there for over a year, but I had never met one particular orthopedic surgeon who was known to be unprofessional and disrespectful to the OR staff. As I walked into an operating room to do his case one afternoon, I felt jerked backward, almost off my feet, by someone grabbing my shirt collar. I immediately spun around and saw a small man, in many respects of the word. Although I am not proud of it, I pushed him into the wall.

"Are you a doctor?" I asked loudly.

"Yes," he replied in a surprised voice.

"Then act like one." I was somewhat embarrassed because I wasn't actually acting much like a professional; I was sinking to his level. The chairman of surgery, however, thought that I acted appropriately to the threat, which, most importantly, didn't affect patient care. The surgeon, however, lost his privileges after my incident was filed along with a long list of complaints against him. The nurses threw a party for me.

I owe that strength to the lessons I learned at camp that year when I met Willie. Willie and I were best friends. I didn't have my own brothers to challenge me physically and mentally. Willie became my brother. We learned that we had a lot in common. Our fathers were both oncologists at the same university. We were both avid tennis players, but weren't good enough to make the team. Both of us loved to snow ski and were frustrated by our East Coast lowlands— we envisioned ourselves as competitive mogul skiers before we even learned how to ski bumps.

Willie inspired me. He seemed fearless. He would somehow sense my fear and encourage me to overcome it. He also added a sense of humor to failing, which made it less scary.

At the top of chair eleven in Vail, overlooking South Rim run, is a fifteen-foot cliff, which takes courage to jump off. One day, Willie and I were following a local ski racer. She flew without hesitation off the cliff, landing into the soft powder, and disappearing into the snow-covered trees below. Willie and I stood atop the cliff. He gave me a look as if to say, "She did it! So can you! Pokin'!" I leapt into the air, and when I hit the snow, my knees barreled into my chest with a loud thump! This was followed by releasing from both skis in what is known as a "yard sale." Anything not firmly attached to me was thrown in a thirty-foot radius. Willie screamed down, "Looks great," and proceeded to jump, producing a yard sale of his own.

There is a fine line between bravery and stupidity. If that cliff jump had ended with an injury, our courage would have been questioned. On the other hand, I didn't want to freeze in the face of fear.

Accepting no risk at all allows for no benefit, known in medicine as "analysis paralysis." It is important to take risks in life, but also to be smart and minimize them when possible. Also, knowing we can bear some pain in our lives strengthens us. Persisting through the pain gives us confidence.

I introduced Willie to his wife. He came with me on one of my first dates with Cheryl. Although we ended up living on opposite coasts, we still lived very similar lives. He is also an anesthesiologist. We have parallel interests, but he always takes his to the next level. We both liked sailboarding, but he would only sail in the thirty-plus knot winds of the Columbia River Gorge. I do mainly indoor rock climbing, while Willie has been known to sleep in a hammock half-way up Half Dome. I guess you could say it's the Parkinson's that held me back, but Willie would never let me think that way (pokin').

WHY I BECAME A DOCTOR

Man never made any material as resilient as the human spirit.
—Bernard Williams

I wish I could say I always wanted to be a doctor. I wish I could say that coming from a long line of physicians meant that my destiny was firmly planted in my mind. I have always said that I ended up a premed major in college because I naturally gravitated toward math and science and struggled with history and English. My story about entering medical school was that I didn't want to find a job, and staying in school was just easier. The truth is I have always had an inner desire to help people. I don't say this to seem selfless. It may well be I wanted that selfish heroic feeling. I don't know for sure. To me, doctors have always had an advantage in health. They know the jargon, the secrets, those "good" doctors. Maybe I wanted to be part of that club.

So I entered medical school, and the first two years were more like intense college. It's not really until the third year that students are exposed to patients, people who are depending on you for help. The third year is when I realized that, as a doctor, I would be able to help a lot of people. But there are limitations, which can be startling. The general public tends to think of doctors as omnipotent. Although it is amazing what we can do, I recall the realization that doctors are human too. I decided to focus on the positive aspects of the field.

I chose a specialty that dealt with acute care. I wanted to see the effects of my treatment right away. I chose anesthesiology because it was just that—the procedures we learned were effective immediately. Usually, I would go home knowing I helped people that day.

I trained in Florida, so because of the average age, there was a lot of heart surgery. I was fascinated by the intensely procedure-oriented fieldof cardiac anesthesiology as well as the fact that we would use the heart-lung machine, which induced a period of suspended animation, while the surgeon worked on the heart.

One patient I assisted just a few years ago stands out in my memory. He epitomized the reason I went into medicine. At eighteen, he didn't know me, nor did he care that I had recently been diagnosed with Parkinson's disease or that I walked funny. He didn't know my name or that I am now retired. He didn't know that I saved his life.

The skies were clear. A huge full moon hung over the US Capitol building during my drive to the hospital that morning. I had been doing that drive for thirteen years before sunrise; never had I seen the moon look so beautiful.

It was a busy day in our heart center. I had just put a patient to sleep for bypass surgery with a senior resident when my partner called for help. An eighteen-year-old male had been brought into MedStar trauma after being shot in the chest on the streets of DC.

As I entered the trauma room, I saw the man on the table looking lifeless. The room had the thick smell of iron created by the copious amount of blood leaving his body and dripping onto the floor. He was so young, probably about the same age as my daughters. I knew instinctively that his parents must have been terrified. I had to professionally push my immediate thoughts away and get straight to work. The young man was cold and limp, and the EKG showed that his heart was making desperate, weak attempts to function as I slipped in an echo probe. Once inserted into the mouth behind the tongue, and down the esophagus like a sword swallower, a transesophageal echo probe sits behind the heart. It gives great ultrasound pictures of the heart, allowing for both diagnosis and more accurate treatment.

Once the echo probe was inserted, I could see that his heart was empty, although it was encased in a high-pressure sac full of blood. He was in cardiac tamponade, which put pressure on the heart from the buildup of fluid.

The young man had been intubated on the street and was getting oxygen, but we had no IV access. We needed to get him a lifeline, somehow inserting a line into his nearly empty vascular system to keep him with us, and we needed to do it fast. I heard the sound of the saw buzzing as the trauma surgeon opened his chest to relieve the pressure. The other doctor, normally calm, now spoke in a high-pitched, fast-cadenced voice. This was somebody's child.

There must have been thirty people in the room for that young man—that child. Our regular, sequenced, balletic team performance had turned into something chaotic and terrifying, something filled with the desperation to save. It was as if all of the doctors were operating on their own son.

With as loud and clear a voice as I could muster, I commanded, "Pass me a central line kit." As I opened the kit and slipped on gloves, I kept my mind on the task at hand. I knew I had to work as quickly as possible; and more importantly, I had to be successful. I had placed this type of line in patients three hundred times per year for the past two decades. I had done this procedure for six thousand people. I knew exactly where the empty vein lived, and had to fight to get there.

A moment later, the sound of my voice seemed to be the only thing in the room. "Line in. Get blood on the rapid infuser." Using a rapid blood transfuser, we were able to quickly replace his blood volume just in time. One of the heart surgeons had also calmly stepped into the room, identified and controlled the bleeder, and stepped out.

The next morning, I went to visit the young shooting victim in the ICU. He was sitting up, reading the sports page. I had been in his trauma operating room for less than ten minutes, and for ten minutes, I didn't have Parkinson's. Or rather, I didn't have the supposed limitations of the disease. There were more important issues to address such as his life. I had a dire purpose in the trauma operating room. His operating room.

That's still how I live my life. Parkinson's disease doesn't define me.

MISDIAGNOSIS

Do not wait for leaders; do it alone, person to person.
—Mother Theresa

To me, my neurological troubles began with a loud boom that threw me forward into the windshield as I was rear-ended by a Cadillac. The driver didn't see I had stopped at a red light, nor did he see the red light. It was 5:30 a.m. in Orlando, Florida, and I was driving to work for a 6:00 a.m. case. I thought I just had whiplash—soft tissue strain without nerve or bone injury. I was thirty-three. It wasn't until three weeks later that I noticed my right shoulder ached, and in general, my right side just felt different from my left.

Sure, I had been rear-ended by a drunk driver on my way to work three weeks earlier, but the car had been fixed, and the accident had mostly slipped out of my mind. I chose to go to a physical medicine and rehabilitation specialist who decided to do trigger-point injections and his own type of physical therapy, which involved passively twisting my neck from side to side. I still shudder when I think about it, because although he didn't know it at the time—but should have—my neck was broken.

This was just the beginning of my journey of misdiagnosis. The physical therapist he sent me to examined me, but refused to touch me until a physician had cleared my neck. An MRI showed a ruptured ligament and protruding disc. I was informed that if a disc protruded in the middle, it implied rupture of the ligament that runs down the back of the spine, which is usually the result of trauma. I thought that was the diagnosis—simple and to the point.

The orthopedic surgeon I saw wasn't sure that a ruptured ligament and spinal cord compression caused my pain, weakness, and foot drop—an annoying condition where I was unable to clear my toes over the floor during a normal walking stride. He wanted to verify the cord compression with nerve conduction studies—tests performed with needles, and only by certain neurologists.

I took my broken neck to a neurologist who did these tests; specifically, nerve conduction studies. They actually measured how fast the impulses traveled along the nerves, and looked for injury or disease. The tests involved needles and electricity, and I didn't like them. This neurologist also wasn't impressed by the MRI, but was impressed by my physical exam. I had increased reflexes, along with other signs of either brain or spinal cord injury. He told me that because I was from the north (Maryland) and had these upper motor neuropathy signs on my exam—meaning a problem with the brain or spinal cord—I most certainly had multiple sclerosis (MS). He then walked out of the room and went home, and I was left alone, wondering what would happen to me. It was exactly as if he had punched me in the solar plexus and left.

Although many people do very well with MS, and live highly productive lives, I didn't know that. He never told me. And I must have been asleep that day in medical school.

In bed that night, I started to cry. I apologized to Cheryl, because she hadn't signed up for all of this. However, she disagreed and told me that she felt that she had. She reminded me of our vows: "in sickness and in health." We cried in each other's arms, and that very act comforted me.

Cheryl has consistently been there for me, an unwavering pillar of strength. Her support alone is empowering. Her medical knowledge is extensive too, and if she doesn't know, she knows someone who does. That's a great marriage—one plus one equals three.

I woke up the next morning with a sense of purpose and a new goal. I decided that I was going to become the world's foremost expert on MS. And if the MS diagnosis was wrong, every minute that passed without decompression would worsen my chance for recovery. I kept in mind that the MRI showed a ruptured disk and broken neck. My back muscles would spasm constantly from trying to protect my spinal cord. The consistent pain kept me grounded and utterly aware.

I soon learned that MS is diagnosed by four tests, three of which are noninvasive. The first is an MRI, looking for areas without the protective myelin sheath that normally covers nerves in the brain. The second is an eye exam, in which an ophthalmologist can see the same areas in the retina. Thirdly, testing the amount of time it took for my brain to receive a signal after a light was flashed in my eyes. While the first three didn't seem so bad, the fourth involved a spinal tap. This surprised me. Why would one remove spinal fluid for analysis when there was already so little due to cord compression? That would only make things worse. I decided to go down the list, starting from the beginning, and saving the inevitable, torturous pain for the end.

I had the MRI, which gave only a ten percent chance of having MS. The next test entailed getting an eye exam. It was Saturday, but I couldn't wait until Monday for results. I called an ophthalmologist who was a friend of mine, and he agreed to meet me at his office. He told me that with ninety percent certainty, he could tell me yes or no to the MS question. My optic nerve was normal. In my mind, if I didn't have MS, then my original diagnosis by the physical therapist was correct, and my spinal cord was waiting to be decompressed. Every hour that went by decreased my chance of full recovery. I was able to get the visual light signal test done that day as well. I began to feel an urgency to find a neurosurgeon.

By Monday, I had completely ruled out MS. I refused the spinal tap. Instead, I was in the office of my favorite neurosurgeon with the spine center at Northwestern, a thousand miles away in Chicago. I had started intravenous steroids at home to protect my spinal cord. I had even started my own IV. The best therapy to avoid further nerve injury while awaiting surgery was IV steroids. Normally, I would have been admitted to a hospital to have an IV started. One of the perks of being married to a doctor is that she could start an IV for me at home. When it came time to start, Cheryl was asleep and I didn't have the heart to wake her. So I just started the IV myself. For the first time, I saw myself on both sides of the needle.

The surgery that I had has a long name. It is called anterior cervical discectomy and fusion. It involved two surgeons. The neurosurgeon took out the ruptured disk, thereby relieving the spinal cord compression. He replaced that space with bone taken from my hip by an orthopedic surgeon. The neurosurgeon confirmed my broken neck, ruptured ligament, and compressed cord. There was some comfort in receiving verification that I wasn't crazy, and that I was right to suspect my diagnosis: I didn't have MS.

It is so important be your own advocate. I think doctors mean well, but as I noticed in medical school, they are human, and medicine is an imperfect science. Don't be afraid to get a second opinion—or a third. Empower yourself with knowledge the best that you can. Luckily for me, I was able to have the stabilizing surgery within four weeks of the original trauma. Even so, my foot drop lasted five years. All this time, I didn't realize my real neurologic challenge was yet to come.

PERSEVERANCE—PART 2

Isolation offered its own form of companionship...
—Jhumpa Lahiri

We were isolated from humanity, from civilization, from the comforts and the stress of society—just the five of us for five weeks. We didn't need cash, electricity or the mail system. As a parent now, I can't imagine the worry that my parents experienced while I was five weeks incommunicado.

It was a pleasure to be in true wilderness, beyond the reach of pollution, crime, and noise. We didn't see another person until we got back to Churchill, Manitoba. We counted on each other.

In that area, the Hudson Bay tide goes in and out for six miles, so you can actually watch it move at one mile an hour. The water was thirty-four degrees. We walked the canoes in the tidal flats at high tide. We were to head next to Eskimo Point, just north of Churchill, where an abandoned Canadian military fort stood. We had planned to stay there on our last night with just the five of us.

Before we could get there, however, we had to portage the canoes the perimeter of a small side bay during high tide, which would have been twenty-two miles. The small bay was aptly named Button Bay. We did have the option of paddling straight across the bay, which would have been a six-mile paddle. We had to consider this very carefully and all be on board as a group. The weather had to be very calm. In the middle, we would be three miles out to sea. We had to be able to see at least six miles to paddle toward the smokestacks of Churchill. Another concern was the frigid water. If we capsized, there was very little chance of survival. Finally, we all knew that Churchill was known as the polar bear capital of the world, and during the summer, adult bears swam the bay looking for food for their young.

The following morning was the calmest we had seen in the bay. We decided to cross, probably because we were tired of walking, and wanted to get paddling again. We used spray skirts to keep water out of the canoes; although with Pitt sitting in the center of our canoe and not paddling, the spray skirt could only cover the bow. In the middle of the supposedly calm sea, we ran into sixteen-foot swells known as non-breaking waves.

Halfway across, Pitt announced, "I'm going to be sick!"

Rory complained that Pitt would capsize us or provide chum for bears. "Pass him a can to throw up in. Pitt, do not lean over the side!"

I passed Pitt a tin can I was keeping to bail water if necessary. Rory instructed Pitt not to throw his puke in the water. I thought it was too late. Over a swell, we noticed four large white animals. Our first thought was that a family of hungry polar bears was following us. As we rode the next swell, we noticed it was a pod of beluga whales escorting us to shore. What a relief! It was as if they were protecting us from bears. They brought us right to the place where the swells became breaking waves, and we had to "ghost ride" the canoes onto the beach. That involved jumping out right and left simultaneously, while supporting the canoes using our legs as outriggers.

We set up camp as planned in the abandoned fort. A couple of hours later, we saw our first human being in weeks. A Canadian Mountie carrying a large rifle approached us on horseback. In a heavy French accent, he said, "It's probably none of my business, but we spotted two polar bears here this morning."

I didn't know what else he said because with that, I flipped a canoe onto my shoulders and ran down to the water! What I didn't realize was that I could have run right into one of the bears napping in the brush nearby! We loaded up our canoes and crossed the

Churchill River, only to find our beluga friends showing us the way again.

We arrived in Churchill three days early. Since we had to wait for our train back to Thompson, Manitoba, we made camp behind a church and made friends with the local Inuit and Eskimos who were very welcoming.

We took a calculated risk that day. We had paddled together for weeks and were a team. We knew each other's capabilities, strengths, and weaknesses, so we went for it without a Plan B. We tackled problems as they arose, using teamwork and experience. The risks remained, but were optimally minimized the best we could. We chose to accept them.

UNANTICIPATED RELIEF

When one door of happiness closes, another opens;
but often we look so long at the closed door that we
do not see the one which has been opened for us.

—Helen Keller

I chose anesthesiology because it was acute; I could arrive in the morning, use my mind, hands, and body to render someone asleep and/or comfortable, and leave at the end of the day as part of a team that had prolonged or maybe even saved a life. The whole team—nurses, techs, attendants, perfusionists, surgeons, surgical assistants, and anesthesiologists—worked together so well that the experience was seamless.

Anesthesiology for cardiac surgery was a highly specialized and rapidly advancing held. Moreover, a certification exam for perioperative transesophageal echocardiography, which is an essential part of the job, had been in place for just two years when I took it. Eventually, all eight of us in our division passed this test.

Training young doctors in anesthesiology residencies in the surrounding area was imperative. With the size of the practice, we always had the necessary clinical load, variety of cases, and enthusiastic physicians; and thus were able to attract residents from two private and three military residencies. We also trained three post-graduate fellows, two of whom went on to start and head their own cardiac anesthesia divisions in medium-sized hospitals in Kentucky and Louisiana.

This was the career I started at thirty-four years old. I was a cardiac anesthesiologist at the Washington Hospital Center, the third-busiest heart surgery center in the country. I worked with the best, most personable, and talented heart surgeons I had ever met. We were truly helping people, and it felt good. That was why I had gone to medical school—to obtain the indescribable feeling of relieving someone of disease and discomfort. Although this was my fourth job as a physician, I knew it was the landing place for my career. I entered that practice in my sixth year out of training. It is said that you learn more in your first five years in practice than all of residency. I was just starting to feel very confident in my specialty. It was thirteen more years before I would begin to lose confidence in my own hands.

I had been clumsy all my life. I remember being twelve years old and playing catcher on the baseball team. I couldn't catch a fly ball to save my life. This worked fine, except for the fact that I had no aim with the ball either, so I often ended up throwing it back over the second baseman's head. Beyond my time playing baseball, there were other differences that separated me from my peers. My walking stride had always been abnormal as if I had to lean forward to get the momentum going, but I always could dance really, really well. Balancing sports like skiing and windsurfing were my thing.

When my neurologist friend examined me and said, "I think I know what's wrong with you," I was relieved. Even before he told me the diagnosis, I felt a weird sense of comfort. Finally, it would have a name. I would now understand this alien feeling I'd struggled with my whole life. I guess I had always wondered why I walked leaning forward, why I always dropped things, and why I couldn't catch a ball—or even throw one.

When he said, "It's Parkinson's," I actually smiled. Now we had a disorder, and we could treat it. I now had a reason to ask for accommodations. Even if I knew only the basics about Parkinson's disease, I knew I would be able to live a full life.

Up until that point, I had only known about the lack of dopamine, the tremors, and the shuffling gait of Parkinson's. I was soon to learn about the stiffness, the slowness, and the freezing.

I asked, "Is it hereditary?"

"Not usually."

"Will it shorten my life?"

"Not usually."

At that point, I could have quit working and used my disability insurance, but after years of training and experience, and only about five years into my dream job, I really didn't want to. My healthy sense of denial served as a great defense mechanism. If I kept life as I normally lived it, then I didn't suffer from Parkinson's. Once I was put on medication that truly worked and felt much better, I was actually bummed because that made my disease harder to deny.

I wish I had learned more about Parkinson's disease in medical school. I think we spent one day on it. The three major symptoms of Parkinson's disease are tremors, stiffness, and slowness. Thus far, it seemed that I was mainly slow and stiff. I learned that the loss of dopamine-producing neurons begins at birth, and once symptomatic, a person has already lost about eighty percent of their *substantia nigra*, the part of the brain responsible for making dopamine. Two out of three people with Parkinson's are male, and ninety percent are diagnosed after age sixty. I wondered why I was lucky enough to be diagnosed in my late thirties.

I understand those with Parkinson's much more now than I ever did. We don't make enough dopamine. Besides being the neurotransmitter responsible for pleasure, dopamine is an inhibitory neurotransmitter in the part of the brain that gives us voluntary movement. Without its presence, we lose finesse and fine motor control. Imagine that your brain is talking to a part of your body with one hundred muscles in it. Your brain says to fire number seventeen only, and dopamine keeps the other ninety-nine muscles quiet. Without it, you have chaotic firing of the nerves for all one hundred muscles at the same time. No good can come of that. Actually, the three main features to Parkinson's disease—slow movement, inability to initiate movement, and tremors—are experienced to varying degrees. Many of us also have no emotion on our faces or fluctuation in our tones of voice. We may actually feel much less emotion as well.

An estimated three million people in the United States have Parkinson's. Only one million have been diagnosed. Although the exact cause of Parkinson's disease is not known, there might be multiple pathways capable of producing the same result. There is even a hereditary type with its own gene mutation. Though I haven't been tested, I am relatively sure mine is not hereditary. I've only had one other relative with Parkinson's disease, my Grandma Bert, and she wasn't diagnosed until her late seventies.

I went back to work that day and called my wife, my parents, my boss, and his boss, and they all had the same reaction to my news of the diagnosis—calmness and confidence I would still live a full life and contribute to society. I had their support.

But I realized that I would need to learn how to ask for help to achieve and maintain a fulfilling life with Parkinson's. This knowledge caused an about-face in life as I had known it before. I had grown up with wonderful role models, and had learned to become independent and autonomous both in my everyday life and in my career as an anesthesiologist. During residency, I initially needed complete guidance; yet by the end of the fourth year, I learned how to do most cases solo. As a resident at this point, I felt very confident on my own, taking things into my own hands. I had been one of two chief residents in a seventy-two-person residency, and my self-worth had become based, in essence, on my ability to know what I needed to know, do what I needed to do, and understand when to ask for help.

Amazingly, through my insidious and worsening coordination and lack of confidence in my own hands, I was still able to intubate and perform the other necessary procedures of anesthesiology with sufficient proficiency to ensure that patients were safe and that residents were being taught correctly.

My competency for those tasks held tight for another ten years, stopping me only when I felt that I couldn't keep working to the high standards I had set for myself.

I told my boss that I didn't feel comfortable working alone as a precaution and commitment to the patients. My division director and chairman had always been incredible as if they had written—or more likely, recently read—the Americans with Disabilities Act. They agreed to support me in any way I needed. I soon stopped taking night calls and was always paired with a senior resident so I could teach with the option of calling for help, if necessary.

Over the next ten years, despite the precautions in place, I never called for help once. In fact, I was still able to show up to help others who needed my assistance.

Possibly, this was because Parkinson's is a disease that occurs at rest rather than in motion. When a person has the motivation and intention to perform a task, anything is possible.

LEAST EXPECTED

Do what you can, with what you have, where you are.
—Theodore Roosevelt

The inability to initiate movement eventually became a major part of my Parkinson's disease. When I can't even begin to move, I look somewhat like a statue or the Tin Man from the Wizard of Oz. I remain frozen in place until I slowly collect dopamine or my meds kick in.

My freezing attacks began four years, post-diagnosis. They were more frustrating than painful and ironically, I would just have to laugh at myself when it happened. It provoked anxiety only if I had someone depending on me; otherwise, I just used comic relief as a defense mechanism. I soon realized that patience was an absolute necessity for this disorder, which didn't blend well with the job of providing anesthesia for heart surgery, requiring the ability to respond swiftly and in a potentially life-saving manner.

The freezing began in a doorway at home. I just couldn't get through the door to my office as if hitting an imaginary wall. My brain simply refused to initiate another step. Once, at a concession stand, I had my drink, popcorn, and change in my hand, but I couldn't walk away. I stood there, completely still, and waited for my brain to reboot. The seller said, "Goodbye!" Thirty seconds later, I walked away.

As we were finishing a case one day, I felt a freeze coming on. My resident wheeled the patient out of the operating room, and I couldn't follow. I collapsed in a chair, twisted at the waist, with one arm up like the Statue of Liberty. I felt like a statue myself.

Surprisingly, I was sitting—if you could call it that—in the operating room for two hours before some attendants decided to return to clean it. Thanks to Carl, an OR attendant—now called Patient Service Attendants/PSA—who was the first to arrive after two hours, I was able to have my meds brought to me. Two hours after that, just as if a light switch had been flipped back on, I regained normal function and drove home without incident.

My chairman caught wind of this and, appropriately, took me out of the operating room. I had seven weeks of paid vacation, and used it to consult with neurologists and adjust my medications to combat the freezing. I was even given a shot that would break the freezing spell. I used it sparingly, though, because it came with two conflicting side effects: nausea and sexual arousal.

During this pause from clinical duty, I continued my resident education and administrative duties, teaching lectures, and making schedules. Although my clinical privileges were on hold, the day came when I had to use them. I was sitting near the back row in a department meeting. There were over forty anesthesiologists in the room, and we were in the process of listening to a long lecture about new rules and regulations when a loud voice came from the back.

"He's down!"

One of my colleagues had collapsed. Instinctively, I jumped over two rows of seats to get to him. Checking for a pulse, I determined quickly that he had a witnessed heart attack. There was no better time to have this happen; forty anesthesiologists had witnessed his heart attack. I pounded him on the chest, and someone handed me a cardiac defibrillator stored in a nearby hospital room.

This defibrillator let me read the rhythm through the paddles that I had applied to his chest. My colleague was in a lethal heart rhythm called ventricular fibrillation. This is a common, treatable rhythm often seen in heart surgery; he couldn't have suffered this type of cardiac arrest in a better place. I shocked him once with the paddles. He came back to sinus rhythm, woke up, and screamed, "Please don't shock me again!"

I don't know if my hunger for work caused me to respond first to this witnessed cardiac arrest—I certainly wasn't the closest to him.

One of the most amazing things about this puzzling disease is that with the right motivation, a person has the ability to move very quickly. My colleague was dying. The movements that I had to make were more reactive than voluntary—they must use a different part of the brain. Sometimes I am frozen, and a simple "come here" gets me moving again. Also, you never hear about Parkies—people with Parkinson's—being stuck in a burning building.

We placed my colleague on a gurney and walked him to the emergency room. We never even started an IV. I guess I was functioning under the Good Samaritan law at that moment. Once we brought him to the ER and he became a patient in the hospital, I was thanked yet reminded that my clinical privileges were still temporarily suspended. Despite this, it felt great to help someone again.

AS BAD AS IT GETS

There is no greater agony than bearing an untold story inside you.
—Maya Angelou

My approach to my new condition was to ignore it at first and hope it would go away. I had been given a seven-week paid involuntary vacation while I waited to see a neurologist at Johns Hopkins to give me the "fit to work" certification. I needed to do something to keep my mind sharp, so I decided to learn to solve the Rubik's Cube. I had recently seen Will Smith do it in a movie, which reminded me that I had always wanted to try that. What I didn't realize was that underneath the meds, my condition was worsening. I had been on meds for five years, and the doses were increasing, and the time between pills decreasing. The relief from the meds was so great that I used to say, "It feels so good when the meds kick in, it's almost worth having the disease!"

Also, I was very sensitive to the negative effects of protein. Certain proteins are known to block the transfer of the meds from the stomach to the brain, and for me, the worst culprits were peanut butter, turkey, and soy. Often I would be frozen by the end of dinner in a sushi restaurant just from the smell of soy sauce. I had never thought about it before, but trying to eat without protein doesn't leave much to eat. I was on a diet of vegetables and crackers. Boy, did I miss cheese! Moreover, my medication dose had gotten so high that I had a ton of involuntary movements as a side effect. I was rapidly losing weight. I really felt as if I was dying.

I treated the medications like a math problem. I figured there was an exact interval between doses that would maximize my therapeutic time and minimize my side effects. I played with it, and finally decided that the perfect dosing interval was two hours and eighteen minutes. I wore a runner's watch, which would alarm every 138 minutes; but of course, this dosing interval didn't remain perfect for very long.

The lowest day in my life was on a weekend. I had lost over fifty pounds, and it hurt to sit down because I had no natural cushion to sit on. Cheryl had bought a "vegetable juicer," and I was trying to drink protein-free celery juice, which tasted like I imagined grass clippings would taste. When I looked in the mirror, I saw an unrecognizable, gaunt, and continuously moving body. Something had to change or I was going to die. I had to think of something.

I knew of a procedure called Deep Brain Stimulation (DBS). I had done the anesthesia for it a few times. I had even seen news stories about people with Parkinson's getting much better with it. With DBS, I could probably take less meds and, therefore, have fewer extra movements. Maybe I would be able to eat protein again.

Here's how it works. A neurosurgeon places an electrical wire into the part of the brain that is not being inhibited well because of the lack of dopamine. From a small pacemaker-like device placed in the chest, a low voltage electrical signal comes out of the end of the wire, and like the squelch on a CB radio, quiets the extra activity so the normal impulses can get through.

This was my only hope. I was desperate.

It was classic thinking in the United States since DBS was approved for Parkinson's a few years after the turn of the century that I first exhausted the medical therapies for PD, and then went to the surgical ones. All surgery carried a risk of complications however low the chance might have been, which was why surgery was the second choice. The truth was that surgery was more effective for a longer period of time with fewer side effects. Most people with DBS said they wished they had gotten it earlier. Because of cost, availability, and the fact that it was surgery, only one percent of those diagnosed with PD underwent DBS.

I saw my neurologist, Dr. Pagan, and asked him if DBS would be a good option for me. He said he thought I would probably be a perfect candidate. First, I had to pass two tests. The first was a dopamine challenge test to make sure that I really had Parkinson's. My dad took me to the hospital for this one. I had to be off my meds completely, and who knew how stiff and contorted I would become? It turned out that my Parkinson's had progressed under the meds, and by the time we got to Georgetown, I was somewhere between a statue and a pretzel. I just had to laugh. As I entered the hospital, one of my former residents was waiting there with a wheelchair. I never found out how he knew I was coming.

I love Dr. Pagan. He is very encouraging and always emphasizes the bright side. He responded that seeing me off my meds since the meds worked so well, DBS should really help me. He had me take the meds right in his office, and watched me unravel and loosen up.

The second test was a neuropsychological evaluation. This was a battery of math and reading tests to test my "executive function." It was like SATs on steroids. They wanted to see how smart I was pre-DBS, so that if my work post-DBS ever came into question, they would have a baseline with which to compare. It showed what I have always known—math skills were great, reading comprehension was not so good.

Math had always come easy to me. This was probably because I had a condition known as synesthesia. The word *synesthesia* refers to the combining of two senses. Usually, it has to do with assigning colors to sights or sounds or smells. For me, I always saw the same colors associated with the same numbers: one-white, two-green, three-orange, four-red, five-blue, six-brown, seven-light green, eight-dark green, nine-pink. It was much easier to remember numbers when they were associated with color.

I thought of letters and days of the week in consistent colors as well. For a long time, I thought everybody did this. So did my daughters who also have synesthesia. In middle school, one of them was reading a book called *A Mango-Shaped Space* in which the main character has synesthesia. They were discussing it at a mother-daughter book club as a rare superpower. Overhearing this, I realized I had a gift.

It was looking pretty clear that I would benefit from getting these wires. I couldn't schedule the surgery soon enough. I researched it in detail. I looked at only centers of excellence (COE) for DBS. The National Parkinson's Foundation has said that if a center has done enough procedures with enough frequency, a high success rate, and low complication rate, it qualifies for this list. They are listed oldest to newest, depending on the date that they obtained the COE status. The oldest on the list was the Cleveland Clinic. I made an appointment to meet their surgeon and learned about what a great preoperative testing system they have. They assigned a patient liaison to meet me in the morning and take me from doctor to doctor as they lined up neurologists, psychiatrists, anesthesiologists, and the neurosurgeon all in one day. It sounded like an impressive system, but actually, I never saw it.

Dr. Pagan sent most of his patients to Dr. Kalhorn at Georgetown, so I opted to look into that facility as well. They also had a COE status for DBS. They had their own anesthesiologist as well as designated physical, occupational, speech therapists, and more. I met with Dr. Kalhorn, and brought Cheryl to see him. We agreed that he was very confident and compassionate. My gut feeling was to go with him and cancel Cleveland. So I did.

WIRED

One who gains strength by overcoming obstacles possesses
the only strength which can overcome adversity.

—Albert Schweitzer

My biggest concern leading up to April 22, 2008, the day I was
scheduled to have my Deep Brain Stimulator implanted, had nothing to do with pain or having a stroke. It had to do with what I was
going to say when they first hooked me up and turned it on. I knew
that whatever I said had to be funny. That was how much trust I had
in my surgeon, my neurologist, and their team. I had heard so many
one-liners, and I had to be original. "I need this like a hole in the
head!" or "It feels like I have my head in a vise!" or "We can rebuild
him."

In the few months prior to the procedure, I was very skinny
because I was always moving. I was taking pills, which had a side
effect of a lot of movement. I was also avoiding protein, and had
gotten to the point where I was almost incapacitated by the disease.
I was desperate for the operation, and anything I said that winter
was related to "when I get my wires." I therefore wasn't worried at all
about complications. It was a Hail Mary. I needed my life back.

I had seen on TV—and even in person a few times—how
DBS got rid of tremors and stiffness, and I had chosen a National
Parkinson's Foundation Center of Excellence for the surgery. It could
only get better from here.

So what was the first thing I was going to say when they first
tested my wires in the operating room and I felt relief? My kids
wanted to know what the plan was too. I ended up borrowing a line

from Radar O'Reilly in *M*A*S*H*, which he delivers as he fixes a radio: "Come in, Tokyo." I thought of my Grandma Bert, who, like me, had Parkinson's disease. We always watched *M*A*S*H* together. "Come in, Tokyo."

This was for you, Grandma Bert.

One thing all Parkies know is that there are three distinct phases we flux in and out of during the day. Without medication, we are *off*, and to us that means we either are moving slowly, frozen, rigid or have a resting tremor. When the meds kick in, it's like a light switch is flipped, and all of sudden we feel normal! If we could somehow stay here, it would be considered a cure. This is why I call that therapeutic window of normalcy "nirvana."

Nirvana lasts only for a short period of time, which actually shrinks the longer we take the meds. It soon transitions into the *over* phase, in which most of us live most of the time. In *over*, the dance-like extra movements become apparent, and we may or may not notice them. We tend to like it here because we are functional. We may look funny, but we can move and do things if we need to. The movements can be annoying, though. Without DBS, it felt like I was always waiting for the meds to kick in or for the dyskinesia—involuntary muscle movements—to go away.

I once described having Parkinson's disease to my daughters as the inability to use all of the little stabilizing muscles most people don't even think about. It's as if the platform from which to move is not even there. Bessie, one of my favorite nurses at work, would see that platform return as I turned *on*, and she would say, "Dr. Lessin, I see you got your gumption back!"

I actually asked for DBS before it was offered to me. After the procedure was completed, I wished I had requested for it even sooner. In my experience, DBS seemed to halt the Parkinson's in its tracks. DBS alone gave me eighty percent of my best *on* time, without causing the extra involuntary movements and spasms. The reason DBS didn't cause those movements was because it was adjustable. If I was flopping around like a seal, I could have simply turned down the amplitude, and the floppiness subsided.

I considered DBS to be an electrical medication that I could adjust. It was a huge aid in taking control of my life. No more waiting to turn *on*, or return from *over*.

I wasn't nervous at all about the procedure. I had complete faith in my surgical team and anesthesiologist, and my faith was always strong. What I was concerned about was the fact that I was supposed to be completely off medication for twelve hours prior to the procedure. Who knew what lay underneath? How stiff would I get?

Cheryl and I decided to stay at the hotel next to Georgetown University Hospital the night prior to the procedure, just to be safe. She was amazing through the whole thing, from diagnosis through treatment. Everyone should have an advocate like her with them when going in for surgery. Knowing she was there for me felt supportive in a way that words cannot describe. Furthermore, she was a surgeon herself, and she was right there by my side, pre-op and post-op. Just try to get into my room without washing your hands!

When I woke up the morning of surgery, immediately I noticed that without meds, my disease had gotten much worse. I could barely move. My body was twisting and contorting into some great yoga poses. I was going to need a wheelchair just to make it into pre-op holding. We called the operating room and asked for a wheelchair, then found out that because we were a hundred feet from hospital property, we needed to call an ambulance. An ambulance for a hundred feet! My wife left for the hospital to "diplomatically" procure a wheelchair. Although she was probably gone for only five minutes, it seemed like much longer.

Lying there alone and curled up like a pretzel, I started to become anxious despite my confidence in the upcoming surgery. Parkinson's symptoms worsen with anxiety, and I started to twist and contort into what I know today as the eagle pose: one thigh crossed over the other, arms parallel with one elbow buried in the crook of another, palms twisted. Getting into this position worsened my anxiety.

I knew I needed to relax and strategize. I raked my mind and then remembered a recent news story about the ability of music to treat Parkinson's disease symptoms. I stiffly pulled out my new iPhone and played a recently downloaded *David Cook's American Idol* video covering the Beatles song "Eleanor Rigby." Almost immediately, it worked. My whole body relaxed despite the contortion. Before the song ended, my wife had returned from her trip, successfully pushing a wheelchair.

Contorting further while being wheeled into the operating room, I started to think that maybe my problem was mainly dystonia, a cousin of Parkinson's, which sustains involuntary muscle contractions and twisting into abnormal postures. It is said that everyone with Parkinson's has dystonia, but the inverse is not necessarily true. I thought it was important to make sure my surgeon saw me without medication, just in case the treatment varied with dystonia. The nurses said I looked so uncomfortable that they got an order for some Ativan to break the dystonia, even though I initially refused it. After a while, I broke down. For forty-five minutes, I sat there in my version of the Bikram yoga eagle pose until my surgeon walked in.

With perfect confidence, he said, "We know what is wrong with you, and we know how to treat you."

It was either his bedside manner or the Ativan, but I immediately felt much more like a champion, and knew I was on track for success.

DBS implantation was a six-hour procedure. The first few hours involved literally having my head put into a vise, although my physician preferred to call it a frame. The purpose of the frame is to provide an exact direction for the wire which, when combined with an exact depth, can place the tip of the wire into a very accurate spot. Once the frame was on, an MRI scan was taken to show the probable target—about the size of a pea. Some surgeons today use a GPS-like device instead of the frame. It has been said that the target is so small that it is like dropping a tennis ball into a swimming pool from thirty thousand feet.

Following the frame, a tester wire was passed deep into the brain using the MRI as a guide. The electrical activity at the end of the wire was played as sound so that everyone in the room could hear. When the wire got to the right place, it immediately sounded like a commotion, lots of chaotic electrical activity that the DBS eventually inhibited. The neurologist then passed a current through this tester wire. This was when they woke me up so I could feel the shackles of Parkinson's lifted from my body. These initial wires were replaced by permanent ones. The whole thing was done under local anesthesia and light sedation.

The fourth-best day of my life began in Operating Room Two at 7:30 in the morning, April 22, 2008. The three best proceeding days were my wedding day and the days my two daughters were born. For the first five hours, I was sedated. I remember nothing. When I woke up for neurological testing, I had the frame attached to my skull, which was surprisingly comfortable. My head was suspended, and my neck felt no pressure. They were working with the tester wires already in place. I could already sense that the procedure was going to be a success. Even with low doses of stimulation, I could feel relief from the chains of my Parkinson's. I could see through his mask that my surgeon had a big smile on his face. That was comforting.

At this point, I felt one discomfort. My bladder was huge. I had to say something.

"I hate to interrupt, but could I get a bladder catheter? Oh, too late!"

I felt the warm urine going down my thighs. Also, I was sitting in a pool of sweat, because I was under a body warmer so I asked for that to be turned off. The next thing I knew, it sounded like a freight train was going right over my head as the next hole was drilled into my skull. That's the last thing I remembered during the surgery. They must have put me back to sleep.

This is the only procedure I am aware of for which a patient must spend the night in the intensive care unit post-op, but can be discharged and go home the following morning. I admit that it was great being the center of attention with my wife by my side and friends coming to visit. That night, I was able to go through the ICU patient experience without being critically ill. I had taken care of many ICU patients during my career, and this was only going to make me a more empathic doctor. Even while recovering from a relatively painless procedure, I had the discomfort of hourly neuro-checks, which involved the nurse waking me to make sure my brain was working. Also, I was feeling a bit like a spaghetti fork with wires everywhere, always in my way.

The highlight of the night was my 3:00 a.m. CAT scan. Many people might consider a CAT scan at that time of day to be a nuisance, but for me it was a "road trip." I got to get out of the confining bed. It felt great to be relieved of the monitors and get into the open air. I'm very grateful to the ICU staff for watching out for me. I gained a better understanding of what it's like to be in ICU for a long time.

Now came the waiting game. I had experienced a taste of what my new wires could do for me during the procedure, but now it would be three weeks before the generator was in place, and another week after that before I would have my new Deep Brain Stimulator turned on for the first time.

Three weeks went by quickly, and I was back in the operating room to have my generator placed. This procedure was to be done under general anesthesia, and I had a little more difficulty after the anesthetic this time. Although I had a wonderful anesthesia staff specializing in neuroanesthesia, I awoke very stiff and unable to move. The amazing thing is that I was discharged from recovery in this condition. I don't find fault with anybody, because until I was a Parkinson's patient myself, I would have done the exact same thing. Being statue-like is a discomfort that doesn't show up on the monitors. We are not trained, as anesthesiologists, to be sensitive to it.

Luckily for me, my father was there, and I was able to convey my discomfort to him. He wheeled me right up to the neurology clinic and found my neurologist who explained to me what was happening. By this time, I had taken more pills than usual by mouth, because they weren't kicking in. Gastric emptying is delayed with general anesthesia. I knew this! My neurologist gave me an under-the-tongue version to break my freezing. I took this to brace myself for the dyskinesia that was on the way from all the pills I had taken. With the new incisions in my chest and head, not to mention the tunneling of wires through my neck, this was going to be fun. My dad brought me home, and for three hours, I lay on the couch flopping about like a Mexican jumping bean. I could only laugh as I simultaneously groaned in pain.

Another ten days went by, and then the moment arrived that I had been looking forward to for months. "Come in, Tokyo!" It was time to turn this thing on.

I was to be off meds once more for this, and I had a one o'clock appointment so my parents brought me to the clinic that morning. We didn't know what being totally *off* would be like for me. My neurosurgeon—once again, the nicest neurosurgeon there is—found me dystonic in the waiting room. He brought me into an exam room with a great view of the football stadium to wait until it was time for my appointment.

By one o'clock, I was a statue. The fellow came in to get me. He said, "Follow me." I thought there was no way I was going to be able to follow him. One of the Parkinson's "bar tricks" is that it can be impossible to actually initiate movement, but when given a command, I can do it. So this Tin Man got up and followed the fellow into the room. He then explained to me that each lead had four contacts, and each contact could be a positive or negative pole. Overall, there were over forty thousand combinations, and with healing during the first year, things would change. He explained that it might take a while to tweak the programming just right.

"Here we go," he said.

He turned it on, and I felt amazing. My whole brain was awake! I felt light as a feather. I jumped up, stretched my arms above my head, and began to run around the clinic. The fellow said, "Come back! I've turned on only one side!"

Over the next nine months, I learned how to adjust the DBS, and met monthly for programming adjustments. On my ninth-month visit, there was a pulse-width change that made a major difference. I had my gumption back. I was alive.

Something about the optimism of the human mind can trick a person into believing that they don't need continuing therapies, because the initial treatment works so well. Sometimes, people feel so good following a procedure that they quickly take for granted the support it took for them to get there. So what does a person in that case often do? They might stop using it, just to see if it's actually necessary, to see if it's critical.

One night, my wife was out of town. I had taken a late pill and felt so good that I turned my DBS amplitude way down while I was still in my office. I went upstairs, then went to bed, leaving my remote downstairs in my office—a mistake I would never make again. At two in the morning, I woke up after the meds had worn off, and could barely move.

I badly needed my stimulator remote and knew exactly where I had left it in my office. I tried to get out of bed, and after about twenty minutes, I slid out, landing face down on the floor. I began to crawl. It probably took me an hour to get to my daughter's door.

"Julie. Julie. Can you get Jimmy on my desk?"

We called the remote Jimmy the Stimmy, followed by my next two DBS remotes, Kimmy and Timmy. The fourth one we called Stanley. Don't ask me why. With a smile, Julie hopped up, jumped over me, and was quickly back with Jimmy. I cranked it up, stood up, and went back to sleep.

FROM THE MOUTHS OF BABES

It's good to have an end to journey toward, but
it's the journey that matters in the end!
—Ursula K. Le Guin

My dad, daughters, and I embarked upon a three-mile hike from my parents' cabin in West Virginia. It was a beautiful fall day, and the forest floor was blanketed in gorgeous shades of brown, red, and orange. Most of our hikes from the cabin led downhill, followed by an uphill return. My parents had bought the highest lot on the hill. I guess they thought it was safer or had better water runoff.

Normally, this wouldn't have been a problem, but one thing I have learned about Parkinson's disease in the last ten years is that it is dynamic. If a person is careful and pays close attention to their body, there is actually a high level of predictability as well. Usually, if I take inventory, I can figure out why I'm randomly stiffening up. It is often a missed dose or a forgotten patch or something. The contrary is also true. Most Parkies have, at least once, felt so good on the meds that we thought we didn't need them. Usually, we found out the hard way that we were wrong.

We had split up into two groups. My father was teaching my younger daughter, Brittany, about milkweed and how to look for bear scat. A few hundred feet ahead, my twelve-year-old and I were about to have a little adventure. We were over a mile from the cabin, and we had at least an hour of dusk and gloaming light before true nightfall.

I felt a freeze coming on. Back then, they didn't give me much warning, and I was always able to attribute them to forgetting a med, having one wear off or eating protein. I stopped in my tracks. It's not as if I was truly paralyzed. I could breathe, and with the right motivation, I could move; but I couldn't voluntarily initiate walking.

The woods were getting dark, and we were without a flashlight. My dad and Brittany were just out of earshot. I had to stay calm. Anxiety would only fuel the fire. My daughter, Julie, was amazingly calm and creative. She remembered that this had happened before, and that I was still able to run or skip; and with this suggestion, I was off. However, I quickly realized that it was going to be tough to run over a mile uphill and in the dark woods.

I don't know how she knew, but she just did. She handed me her walking stick, and I put it up behind my neck like an ox yoke. She had seen me do similar things before over the years, and she had remembered subconsciously that doing this same maneuver with ski poles had helped in the past. I have no idea why it works, but it does. With it, I miraculously was able to walk. Years later, I realized that she had understood my voice and situation when no one else would have been able to.

My daughters are each fantastic in their own way, but I am not sure how much of that we, as parents, can take credit for. Although they depend on me less and less as they age, they still know they can rely on me. In many ways, Parkinson's disease reverses this dependency so they were asked to grow up at a young age. My children, who were supposed to be counting on me, often ended up providing the support I personally needed.

My younger daughter is full of life and, like yoga chi, shares her energy with me via laughter, which is better than any medicine. In the days before DBS, I used to freeze almost every night, because I would let the meds wear off. My second daughter was fascinated with our work as physicians, and she would come running in, screaming, "Good! I get to give him a shot!" I would start laughing uncontrollably as my fourth-grader picked up the injector, saying, "How do you use this thing?"

Humor and the ability to laugh at my own situation felt fantastic. I would get "attacked" every morning at breakfast when my early meds kicked in. My right arm and leg flopped around, while my left side remained totally functional. My family became so used to it that I could be driving a car, and they wouldn't even notice. I'd cure it in thirty seconds by turning down my DBS on that side.

I was showing off one morning as I said, "Here it comes!" and preemptively turned down my stimulator, only to be immediately halted like the Tin Man in Oz.

Without skipping a beat, my daughter said sarcastically, "You weren't getting attacked, were you, Daddy? Now you gotta turn it back up!"

Laughing at my own situation made it seem far less serious.

I can only hope that my disease has not had a negative impact on my daughters. They both have known me only since I've had symptomatic PD. Sure, they have seen videos of the younger, more coordinated, faster-moving Dad. However, the person they see every day is more introverted and less energetic. My temper is on a shorter fuse. Even so, they seem to understand me very well. Possibly, my Parkinson's has made them more sensitive, understanding, and patient. Maybe I can't take credit for that, and they are just two wonderful kids.

TWO-WHEELED THERAPY

Nothing compares to the simple pleasure of a bike ride.
—John F. Kennedy

I had always loved riding a bike, but had never considered myself a cyclist. Even today, when I get on my bike, the side effects of my Parkinson's seem to vanish for the most part. Ever since I was a kid, I've always had a mountain bike, and used to love to ride the single-track trails while living in Jacksonville, Florida in the mid-1990s. More recently, prior to my DBS, I had put courier tires on it, and would ride a local trail for about a twenty-mile loop.

Six days after my DBS was turned on, I was back on my bike. I was so happy to be alive and able to enjoy being outside that I would loudly say, "Good morning!" to everyone I encountered.

I must have had a big smile on my face, because I overheard somebody say, "Here comes that happy, good morning biker!" I was just amazed that I could actually ride.

About three months after DBS surgery, I was sitting on the couch watching the Beijing Olympics. Taylor Phinney had achieved seventh place in cycling, and they had a color story on his father, Davis Phinney. Davis is a super-successful American cyclist, having won the Tour de France stages in the mid-1980s. He had been diagnosed with Parkinson's disease about five years earlier, and had just recently received DBS. He got his DBS a month before I did, and was talking about how his Parkinson's symptoms got better with cycling.

This wasn't the first time I had heard of this. A neurologist at Cleveland Clinic decided to bring one of his Parkinson's patients along on a tandem bike for a one hundred-fifty-mile ride. At every rest stop, the patient would try to do the grapevine—well known to soccer players as a sideways crisscross warm-up maneuver—and he would feel better and better as the ride went on. The theory is that being forced to do rapid, alternating movements like pedaling a bike causes the brain to produce dopamine. This may explain why I have always felt better on a bicycle.

That was the first day I realized that I needed to exercise if I was going to live my best with Parkinson's. I got up off the couch, drove to the bike shop, and bought a road bike. This new bike was lighter and had bigger wheels than my old mountain bike. My goal was to ride one thousand miles in the first year, and I decided to do it to benefit the Davis Phinney Foundation. I recorded the miles on a computer, and would ride almost daily. I felt good when I was riding, and even better about two hours after I finished. I rode three thousand miles in that first year, and it was all because of The Spartans.

The Spartans is the name of an amateur cycling group made of up middle-aged men and a couple of women, which I founded with two friends. I first saw Bruce's new bright-orange Fuji bicycle at our daughters' soccer game. I asked Bruce if he wanted to ride together, and he offered to meet at my house on a Saturday morning. Bruce showed up on a steel Spalding bike that he had found in his neighbor's trash—in basketball shorts, sneakers, and no helmet.

We started down my usual trail, and Bruce was quickly going twenty-two miles per hour, which is pretty fast for us amateurs. I was just wondering how I was going to hold this pace when he bonked, which is a biking term for "loss of energy." I blew by him with ease. This surprised me, because Bruce is now known as "Juice." He was one of the fastest, strongest, and most consistent Spartans. He was also always the first rider to voluntarily hang back with one of us who was struggling.

During those first few rides, I would make it back up the hill about ten minutes before Bruce with enough time to have a snow cone, waiting for him upon his return. Bruce eventually invited another school parent, Michael, to join us, and this was the real start of The Spartans.

Michael, who named the team, was extremely good on hills because of the Irish quads he inherited from his father, so we quickly nicknamed him "Crush." My nickname came shortly afterward.

They called me "Mash," because someone with Parkinson's disease pedaled more slowly in a higher gear. I was a masher.

The Spartans grew quickly through word of mouth. It didn't take long before we added others, like Doc, Teach, Magic, Spin, Quiet Storm, and many more. We were excited when we discovered that we had an e-mail list of forty riders meeting every Saturday morning for a standard twenty-eight-mile ride, which included one big hill halfway through. At first, we simply called it "The Hill."

On a bike, I could actually stay with the middle group. We generally kept a pace of sixteen to eighteen miles per hour on the flat part of the ride on the way to The Hill. I noticed that my mood, and self-worth for the coming week, correlated with what place I came in on that hill. I would pedal as hard as I possibly could for that one mile of average six-percent grade, and would usually end up somewhere in the middle.

Each week, there would always be some new riders who were not yet in shape and would fall behind the pack. A handful of times, I came in first, second or third, but nobody ever beat Crush up the hill that now bears his name: Fitz Hill. I was always happy as long as I gave it my all and left nothing out on that hill.

I think it's unreal that a guy with Parkinson's can, in his mind, compete with the neuro-intact or people without the disease. This is when I first realized that although Parkinson's is a dynamic situation, during certain *on* times and with the proper DBS adjustment, I can be surprised by what I am able to accomplish.

The other unspoken competition inherent to the group had to do with equipment. Each week, we would show up at 7:30 a.m. in the parking lot and notice any new piece of equipment. It would usually be something lighter, and therefore more expensive. The following week, a few more of us would have the same thing. I find it ironic that we all enjoy the workout of cycling, yet we buy gear to make the ride easier and shorter. I ended up with carbon everything, which is the lightest material used. I needed all the help I could get.

Of course, in the era of social media, we soon created a group webpage, and the e-mail banter became the best part of the weekly Spartan experience.

From the Juice:

10/15/2009; 2:33 p.m.

I'd been meaning to put this e-mail out earlier this week, thanking the two riders who rode with me last Saturday. If you could have seen my face when I arrived where we meet each Saturday-I was pitiful. I looked like a man without a friend.

No Mash, no Teach, no Quiet Storm, no Kim (okay, she never shows up). No Jag.

Not even a last-minute call from someone saying they could not make it- it was bad! As my church-going mother would say, "God is good!" Like a knight with a cool-axx bike, my man (Mufasa) did not let me down! Riders-please welcome Mufasa to the group. Dre and I started down the path (you know the path). Out in the distance, I saw a man, sitting on top of a park bench adjusting his gloves as though he was a world class fighter about to destroy his enemy. It was him-my other partner in crime, The King Of The Hill! (Crush). Thank you, man. Needless to say, we had a great ride, and I saw the enemy (the Hill)-and he destroyed it!

I missed that ride, but went out the next weekend. This time, I wasn't so lucky.

From the Masher:

10/17/2009; 9:58 a.m.

Just returned from the ride. You should have seen the Masher, pulling into the parking lot at seven-thirty, alone, not a friend in the world. No Juice, no Crusher, no... well, you know who you are. My mother never even went to church; she's Jewish. I waited for Mufasa, the Garmin salesman... nothin'. I hit the trail (same one as in Juice's story) and as I crested the hill and looked at the empty Mass Ave. bench, I shed a tear (actually, it was just a drop of rain) because I knew one thing... I was going to be first up that hill today!! I rode on... one man and a bike... alone with his own thoughts (scary), and so in my head, for twenty-eight miles, I wrote this blog. I did find God as I prayed not to fall on the switchback (both ways). I am home without a scratch, and my toes are regaining their feeling right about now. Clothes going in the dryer, and I will seey' all in the a.m.!

Here's an e-mail that sums up just how important cycling and The Spartans are to my living well daily with Parkinson's disease:

10/15/2010

I was on my trainer just now, facing the man in the mirror, and I started thinking that without biking and the Spartans (and my stimulator) I would be in rough shape. So at the risk of Juice "kickin' me in the shins!" I wanna get sappy for only a quick second.

Thank you!!!! Thank you to all of the Spartans, as you inspire me to ride and keep rollin'. Each of you has been encouraging, and has stayed back once or twice when I couldn't get it right.

Maybe because I was one of the groups founders, but all of the Spartans have always been good to me. Parkinsons follows the law of physics: a body at rest tends to stay at rest, and a body in motion tends to stay in motion. More simply put, if you don't move, you won't move. I found out early that the more I exercise, the better I feel, so I've tried to find safe and effective ways of tricking my brain into producing more dopamine—if that's what it's really doing. Cycling is one of them.

I realize that I've tried countless things I never would have considered without the diagnosis of Parkinson's disease. A person has to prove to himself or herself that they can do it. With the Spartans, I ended up riding two century rides (one hundred miles), and four one hundred-hfty-mile, two-day rides. With a team, a person can push faster and travel farther. As part of a group, a person is definitely stronger than the sum of their physiology. That whole "one plus one equals three" thing. The second day of the first MS 150, we figured that out.

> 5/23/2010; 7:58 p.m.
> It was beautiful.
> It followed a Saturday of our usual—going all-out, all the time—with most of us cramping up around mile fifty, and finishing in three or four small groups.
> Sunday, it happened: the Spartans became a team. All egos were put aside, and our most important goal became staying together as a team, supporting each other, and finishing as one tight group. We decided first thing in the morning that we were going to ride as a team and leave no Spartan behind. The Mav came up with a fantastic communication method to make sure we were all together and tight. It would also identify if anyone was limping. We never passed each other, and the puller would peel off and go all the way to the back and count the team to make sure we were all there. The ride was seventy-five miles of efficient Spartan machine. We crossed the finish line as a team, all together.

I want to give a special thanks to all the Spartans—especially the Juice, who was behind me when I stiffened up during the seven miles before lunch. Everyone "tightened up" for me, and Juice was very supportive.

We saw the advantage of a pace line. A very enjoyable ride. We are a team.

"Eight Strong!

SLOPES

Nothing is impossible, the word itself says, "I'm possible!"
—Audrey Hepburn

I have been skiing almost as long as I have been walking. For some reason—which we now know—I have more grace on a pair of snow skis. Also, for as long as I can remember, I have always felt very comfortable snow skiing. I have not let a winter go by without strapping on a pair of snow skis.

When I was a young boy, my family would all load into the Vista Cruiser and join my aunts, uncles, and cousins in the Upper Peninsula, Michigan, for a week of subzero skiing. We would stay in an A-frame cabin at Big Powderhorn Lodge. I have wonderful memories from those winter family vacations.

When I was a young teenager, my dad took me to Keystone, Colorado, and I fell in love with the Rocky Mountains. The weather was warmer, the snow was better, and the runs were longer. Not to mention the fact that the scenery was breathtaking! After that, I successfully bargained with my dad to move the family ski trips out west.

At age sixteen, my best friend, Willie, and I went out to Snowbird, Utah, with the sole purpose of learning how to ski the bumps. Also known as mogul skiing, it required a lot of leg and core strength, fast agile movements, and a little fearlessness. We found the perfect run to ski repeatedly for practice. Lower Primrose Path had small round moguls with the perfect pitch to learn on. Moguls are bumps in the snow formed by skiers in a way that if one skis between the moguls, they pass alternatively on the right and the left. As we learned to ski them faster, we needed to move our feet faster from side to side to check our speed on the moguls and retain control.

There was a nine-minute chairlift over Lower Primrose. The run took about six minutes downhill. We would ski this same run over and over, about four times an hour, from the lift, opening to closing time for the entire week. Willie and I learned to ski moguls that week, but it would be a run in Vail, Colorado that we spent most of our ski time in the bumps for the next fifteen years.

In my teens, there was one (and only one) run that I wanted to ski. Highline in Vail is literally a mile of moguls. It's never groomed, and it's just the right pitch to form beautiful bumps resembling large scoops of ice cream. We would ski this run ten to twenty times in a row until my back and legs were so sore that I could barely walk to dinner unassisted.

I loved that run. I continue to take an annual trip to Vail, gravitating toward that bucket of bumps. There was a period before I was wired when I would have lots of trouble on the moguls, tire quickly, and find it impossible to turn right. My answer to that was to just quit turning, so I would end up skiing straight—very fast and close to the trees on the left-hand side of the run. Eventually, the sound of trees whizzing past my head inspired me to buy a helmet.

One of the most amazing examples of the beauty of DBS became apparent my first time back on Highline, after I got my wires. I couldn't believe it! I skied it like I was twenty-five again! Of course, I could ski it only once, because I was physically spent afterward— but I could turn right and left quickly and ski a line of bumps, just like I used to. I was so excited that I surprised two strangers I shared the chairlift with. "I have to tell you guys something. I just skied my first Highline after getting my brain pacemaker for Parkinson's, and the difference is incredible! It's like twenty years ago!"

As it turned out, coincidentally, one of them was a nurse, and she knew exactly what I was talking about.

I was back in the bumps. It never ceases to amaze me what a Tin Man can do with the right motivation.

PERSEVERANCE—PART 3

I'm not in this world to live up to your expectations
and you're not in this world to live up to mine.

—Bruce Lee

As an adult, I realize that my Canadian canoe trip at age sixteen was not only a lesson in perseverance, but also a challenge to persist in the face of overwhelming fear. Rory, our fearless leader—literally or so it seemed—would show us the lakeside cliffs formed by the glaciers' edges. When they receded, they left behind cliffs along the lakes edge, perfect for jumping into the deep fresh water at their bases. The few seconds of freefall seemed like eternal bliss, immensely exhilarating.

Rory had been excitedly talking about cliff jumping from the beginning of the trip. Our first jump was as a group on the drive up to Wollaston Lake, Saskatchewan. It was off a thirty-foot bridge, and into the fast-moving Churchill River below. The fast water created less surface tension, so there would be less of a jolt when one's boots smacked into the surface. This was supposed to be a "good luck" jump.

I have never really been a believer in luck. However, somebody from one of the other groups refused to jump.

Unfortunately, two weeks into the trip, their group had tipped both canoes in a gorge and they lost all their gear, leaving one of them, the non-jumper, clinging to a rock in the rivers center. He quickly became hypothermic. They needed a miracle, but miracles seemed to be mythical. But just then, as if their bad luck had run out, a rarely seen supply helicopter showed up on its way to a northern gold mine. All of the members in that group were rescued and brought to the mine, where they gladly and gratefully worked for their keep as our camp sent a van for them.

Unlike that group, our group had all jumped off the bridge and swum diagonal to the current to get us right to shore without incident. Over the next few days, we would see the hieroglyphic-covered cliffs tempting and taunting us. We wondered when we were going to jump again.

The best cliff was on Bear Lake where we camped for a day, and jumped off a forty-foot cliff about a dozen times. This really brought our cliff-jumping confidence up. Later in the trip, we would discover that forty feet was fun and slightly anxiety provoking, sixty feet was very anxiety provoking and only slightly fun, and eighty feet was simultaneously terrifying and not worth it.

The eighty-foot cliff, as labeled on the map, arrived right at the end of the Cochrane River Lake Chain. We had been anxiously anticipating it during the days proceeding. We parked our canoes, then climbed up the side of this mammoth rock formation; the lake below began to look farther and farther away. Eventually, the view was similar to looking out of an airplane on approach. My heart raced; I had this sinking feeling in my stomach, because I knew I was making a big mistake. This cliff was too high and we were in the middle of the wilderness. I really didn't want to do this.

Rory insisted that he would jump first to ensure its safety. Although we had swum all around the landing zone, assuring there were no submerged boulders, the first jumper was most likely to find out about missed ones or rock protrusions in the cliff that we didn't notice.

I insisted on jumping second for a much less intelligent reason: I just wanted to get it over with. As I looked over the edge of the cliff, I took a deep breath, and with a running start, flung myself over the ledge. It seemed like I was falling for eternity. I tried to keep my boots down, but that was a huge struggle. After an actual three or four seconds of falling, I hit the water hard and slightly off axis. This knocked the wind out of me. I sank quickly, about twenty feet or more beneath the surface. My lungs were empty from screaming the whole way down, so when I finally emerged back on the surface, I was starved for air. For a few seconds, I thought the landing might have actually injured me. Trying to catch my breath was excruciating. Rory had to help me swim to shore. Luckily, as I calmed down, I was able to catch my breath. I'm never doing that again!

I was surprised that Pitt and Watt jumped right behind me, completely unscathed. Fred was the only smart one, proving to be the most mature of us all. He didn't succumb to peer pressure to leap off the cliff and take the eighty-foot plunge to the frigid water below. He decided not to jump. I thought about this moment several times as I grew older and matured. I didn't need to jump. I realized that didn't just apply to jumping off cliffs into massive bodies of water but to life in general. Fred is the one I should thank for many decisions I have made later in life, especially with my Parkinson's. Although I have to continually push myself and find my new boundaries, I have to do it safely, knowing that I am living with a new set of limitations. There's one question this experience has left me with that shaped up my life: Is it really worth it?

RIDING THE ROCKIES

Life is like riding a bicycle. To keep your
balance, you must keep moving.
—Albert Einstein

In my rearview mirror, I saw the flashing red lights of the Maryland State Police. I knew he was looking for me. I was so exhausted that I was struggling to stay in my lane. I had just finished my last century (hundred-mile) ride, which was very tough for me. After that ride, I was so drained that I found it difficult to stay awake on the drive home. It must have been obvious to other motorists, because I was eventually pulled over by a very nice police officer who instructed me to take a mandatory one-hour nap, while he stayed parked next to me. I swore I would never do another long ride again.

I realized that it could be exceedingly tricky to keep my meds and my stimulator adjusted so that I would be able to pedal effortlessly. Usually, on those long rides, I would feel great for the first ten miles, then I would seem to lose the ability to turn the pedals over quickly. During the second half of that particular century ride, the headwinds kicked up to thirty-five miles per hour, which only added to my challenge. It was all I could do to maintain six miles per hour as I struggled to finish the last ten miles. What should have taken forty minutes became a two-hour push into a wind tunnel worse than any hill.

I finished that century ride with three Spartans who had decided our teamwork was most important, and stuck close to the motto "no Spartan left behind."

Six months later, I was invited by the Davis Phinney Foundation to join them for an anticipated four hundred-fifty-mile ride over seven days with other Parkies across the Colorado Rockies. Following my encounter with the police officer, naturally, I was hesitant to accept. Ignoring driving afterward, biking four hundred-fifty miles sounded like an insurmountable idea. How was I ever going to average seventy-five miles per day for seven days straight?

Even though it seemed impossible, raising money for the Davis Phinney Foundation was definitely a plus. This foundation not only supports Parkinson's disease research; it also supports caregivers, and promotes exercise for Parkinson's disease therapy. In their mission statement, they discuss the idea of celebrating the small victories, and living well with Parkinson's. They are not just waiting for a cure. They are assuring us that we can work with what we have today, and that as long as we move, we will stay in motion.

SAG (support and gear) is a three-letter acronym in cycling which refers to the people who look out for the cyclists, and help them with food, drink, and mechanical support if needed. The only way that I would even consider riding this crazy ride is with my own personal SAG buddy. I called Dan—we Spartans called him Amtrak. This was going to be an extremely physically challenging ordeal, and to be safe, I needed to have someone behind me on a bike looking out for me. Dan and I had been friends since medical school. I was in his wedding, and he was in mine. Dan is definitely the type of person I refer to as a two-in-the-morning type of friend, someone you can call at any time of the day or night who would drive or, in Dan's case, fly in a small, private plane to help you without question. I offered Amtrak the SAG job, and he took it without hesitation.

We began to train for Ride the Rockies (RTR) about three months before the ride. In my mind, we were training for altitude and climbs. In Maryland, we have neither. We do have a mountain, Sugarloaf, which towers 1,200 feet above sea level and features three miles of climbing. For training purposes, we soon determined that this was the closest we were going to get to the Rocky Mountains. We learned a very good route. Actually, the approach to and return from Sugarloaf had more ups and downs than the actual mountain. We met for seven Wednesdays, embarking on the forty-four-mile trek by 9:30 a.m., returning earlier and earlier each time.

Every Wednesday, we met in a parking lot at a swim center and pedaled the twenty-two miles out to Sugarloaf. On weekends, we were on our own for endurance work. The midweek ride was mostly through neighborhood streets, and it was anything but flat. For four and a half miles, we pedaled alongside Route 28 with a speed limit of fifty-five miles per hour. I would just pray for those twenty minutes that we wouldn't be the victims of a distracted driver. A good friend of mine, known as Puller, a year earlier had been hit by a fast-moving school bus on that same stretch of road. Amazingly, after major surgery and six weeks in a medically induced coma, he lived to ride again. As I passed that spot each week, I would say a little prayer thanking God for his good fortune. We also had good fortune. It never rained, we gained endurance, and learned how to relax and "settle in" during a climb.

Parkinson's disease added two more dimensions to the elements we needed to cycle effectively. Neurologically intact bikers generally are concerned with aerobic fitness, flexibility, nutrition, and hydration as primary factors. I had to add timing of medication and adjusting the amplitude of my DBS to the mix. During my training rides, per my neurologist's suggestion, I added caffeine as a rescue drug. I added a small bottle of five-hour Energy, with less caffeine than a cup of coffee, to my water bottle, and took another bottle with me. It worked faster than the Levodopa pills when Parkinson's disease threw the chains on during the ride, and I could actually feel my brain gather its gumption. My legs could spin again!

During one of the early Wednesdays, I was slowing down about halfway through, and a pickup truck pulled up next to me to cheer me on. Unfortunately, the truck got a little too close to me, and since there was no shoulder, I dove into a roadside ditch. Dan had gone on ahead of me, and had probably pedaled about three extra miles by the time he realized I was no longer behind him. He had to circle back to find me, sitting on the side of the ditch and pulling grass out of my shifters. Dan must have vowed to stay behind me and never pass, because after that, he was reliably there. It can be much more difficult to climb a hill or even descend at a slower pace than would normally feel natural to you, because to maintain that slower pace requires a harder gear, and quad burn will set in earlier. Dan never complained.

I boxed and shipped the bikes to Telluride, Colorado, two weeks before the start of Ride the Rockies. While I waited for the calendar to change, I learned that there would be two thousand riders total in Ride the Rockies; twenty of us represented the Davis Phinney Foundation group. The ten riders I had expected with Parkinson's disease had been reduced to three, one of whom would be on a tandem bike. Only one other fellow Parkie was riding solo. I reached out to her by phone, and found out she was a local Coloradoan who rode those mountains all the time.

Dan reassured me that we would pace ourselves wisely on this challenging ride and enjoy the mountain views. I had developed a philosophy, which I had displayed on my mantel at home on a piece of wood carved with that quote I used to describe my philosophy about cycling and life: "Life's not a sprint; enjoy the ride."

And I did.

It was an all-day affair to get us out to Telluride. It was late spring, the snow had recently melted, and all of the wildflowers were in bloom. It was as if the wildflowers were meant to lead us on the seven-hour bus ride toward the most physically challenging week of my life. We were nervous and excited. We noticed that most of the riders were middle-aged men, like us. It seemed that this group also wanted to challenge themselves, just to prove that they could still do so.

We arrived to find our bikes there. Great news found its way to my cell phone while I unpacked and got ready for the next day. It was a text from my wife. "This is your named award." There was a picture of a crystal trophy inscribed, "The Lessin Award. For Inspirational Leadership in Perioperative Care." This was wonderful—the perfect psychological boost I needed right at that moment. I had known that I was going to miss the Georgetown Anesthesiology residents' graduation. I had requested that my wife accept the award on my behalf. I thought it was going to be a standard teaching award, which would have been more than enough. These wonderful young doctors had recognized me in a way that confirmed the validity of my continuing to work for as long as I did. My teaching had been appreciated. This feeling of confidence somehow morphed into my cycling psyche, carrying me through the next seven days.

The next morning, we woke before the sun rose and tried to get an early start. My fellow Parkie, Margaret, met us out in front of the hotel with her sister and SAG buddy, Beth. Beth knew the area, she knew the drill, and she had a car. Being a triathlete, she could easily have ridden with us, but her decision to keep close by with her car turned out to be indispensable.

After a lot of administrative dealings, and a lot of breakfast for Dan—he would soon earn the name "Flapjack Dan"—we were off. The first day gave us a taste of what the rest of the ride would be like. Each day included a major climb, usually in the morning, followed by a long descent. The ride was laid out on the map by elevation, which ranged between six thousand and eleven thousand feet. It appeared that days three, six, and seven had no pass to climb. Like a wolf in sheep's clothing, they turned out to be our hardest days.

On the opening day, we traveled from Telluride to Cortez. Right out of the blocks, we climbed Lizard Head Pass. I quickly learned how to sit back and settle in for that five miles uphill. In my mind, I repeated the mantra, "Sit down, relax, breathe." I tried not to hear the other voice in my head that said, "Ignore the pain in your legs, the burning sweat in your eyes, the hunger for air, the guy behind you who wants to pass!" Settling in is more mental than physical. It may seem obvious, but it bears saying that only helpful thoughts are helpful. My meds kicked in for the last mile, which I know made Dan happy, because we must have passed a hundred riders before we reached the top.

There, I met Connie Carpenter, the wife of Davis Phinney, for the first time. I just had to tell her how moved I had been by a story I had read online about her son, Taylor Phinney, *This Is Not a Story About Last Place*. The article described an Italian professional race in which Taylor, a world-class cyclist, was suffering after being dropped into severe weather conditions, including high winds and freezing rain, which had caused most of the pack to quit the race. Taylor persisted for hours in the cold, wet conditions, and he was able to ride up the twenty-two-percent-grade hills because he was thinking only about his dad. More specifically, he was thinking that his dad would gladly have been out there in those conditions if it meant that for one day, he could be free of Parkinson's disease. After reading that article, I found myself in tears, and wrote to the Davis Phinney Foundation:

> My sister-in-law put this story on my fb, and it is the most amazing, inspiring story I have ever read. I don't know if it's because I am a cyclist, a father, or a fellow YOPDer, but I haven't stopped crying for an hour (in a good way!). Taylor has the heart of a lion and an immense love for his dad that is very touching. Now, more than ever, I am honored to be riding for the Davis Phinney Foundation in June.

That night, at dinner, my daughter read the story to my family, and the floodgates opened again.

After Lizard Head Pass, we had discovered how amazingly far a person could go downhill in the Rocky Mountains. We were up a half-mile long, but manageable, climb at only four percent grade by nine o'clock that morning. The entire rest of the day was literally a coast downhill, dropping from eleven thousand to five thousand feet over the course of thirty miles.

I posted this Facebook entry after the second day:

> Two days, one hundred forty miles into Ride the Rockies! Met Bob Roll—a Tour de France commentator—at dinner tonight. This ride has the longest climbs and descents I've ever seen. Getting it all on GoPro. In Durango now to Pagosa Springs tomorrow. Looking forward to the hot springs. Dan and I are riding well.

I don't know why, but I decided to utilize the free bike tune-up service after the second day. That's when the mechanic told me how lucky I was. A crucial part holding the chain taut on the back of the bike was hanging by a thread. "If this thing called a derailleur hanger had come off, and gone into the spokes on the descent, the wheel would have locked up and—" I stopped listening. I couldn't allow myself to worry about "could haves" that didn't happen. I had enough "dids" to worry about.

This was actually a blessing in disguise. Since they had to keep my bike for a day while waiting for a part to be shipped, I rode a loaner bike with a better gear ratio made for climbing hills. What I didn't know was how thankful I was going to be to be riding that climber the next day.

The third day looked easy on the map. It was only eighty-four miles, and Hesperus Hill had to be easier to climb then a mountain pass. I learned that day that the only factor that differentiates a pass from a hill is that a pass is actually lower than its surrounding area, whereas a hill arises out of lower land. This proved to be a very physically challenging day. We climbed the entire time. It was amazing to me how much I could drink and still feel thirsty. I think I had four cans of Mountain Dew, four large smoothies, and eight water bottles full of Gatorade that day. At about mile fifty, Dan and I flagged down the water guy as he passed, to drink and refill. He was a gift. That day featured a paucity of shady trees, and at one point, we found ourselves sharing the shade of a lone ponderosa pine with about twenty cyclists.

Today was the hardest day, I think. Day three. Eighty-four miles, but the last thirty miles uphill on tired legs. Tomorrow we climb first thing fresh for twenty miles, and the next seventy-one are downhill. We peak at Wolf Creek Pass at ten thousand, five hundred feet. I'll let you know how it goes.

Every day, I had my DBS to thank for the fact that I was able to hop out of bed in the hotel room, and get on the bike at six in the morning. Our nights were all the same. I would get to the Davis Phinney tent, and they would usually have chocolate milk waiting for me. I would then ride to the hotel and collapse on the bed, in full cycling garb. I wasn't sure if I was able to move or not, because I would immediately fall asleep, awakening two hours later to the sound of my buddy Dan bringing in my bags.

I would summon enough energy to grab a burger somewhere, then head straight back to the room. Usually, as I stared at the bed I couldn't wait to get into, I would spend about an hour making sure my equipment was ready for the next day. Once clothes, meds, bike, and camera were organized, I would hit the sheets. By this time, Dan would be lying on his bed fully dressed, iPad on his lap as he attempted to watch Netflix, but he always fell asleep after the first five minutes of the movie. Like clockwork, at about midnight, I would chuckle as I heard him wake up and say, "Damn! Not again!"

We had been waiting for the arrival of Wolf Creek Pass. I had to get my gumption up for day four. Climbing out of Pagosa Springs in a single-file serpentine of cyclists, ascending eight miles into the clouds, was very intimidating for this East Coaster. Because I am a "masher," I carry an extra-large, fifty-five-tooth chain ring on the front, so my small front ring isn't actually that small. This can make climbing more difficult. To add to the fun, the average grade on this ascent was eight percent, and even the tractor-trailers were moaning as they struggled up the Wolf.

As Amtrak and I settled into our lowest gear, I made a plan that we would pull over and stop every two miles. Before we knew it, we were at a beautiful scenic overlook with the first two miles behind us. The next six didn't come quite so easily. Pretty soon, we were stopping every half-mile, then every quarter-mile. I would like to say it was the altitude that was causing air hunger, but I think it was the maximum physical exertion! The peak that morning was eleven thousand feet, and when we arrived at the rest stop up top, I was elated. Dan was too, because they had his favorite meal of the day for The Flapjack Guy.

Five days down, four-hundred-ten miles behind me. We've climbed almost fifteen thousand feet. Three passes and huge descents. Tomorrows route is now ninety-four miles to avoid the wildfires. They have added four thousand, five hundred feet of climbing to the ride. I'm doing well. I'll keep you posted.

The Flapjack Guy had his own pancake-making system. He had a griddle and had built a machine on an axis that could squirt out four pancakes at a time, starting with either two or four flapjacks, complete with lots of butter and maple syrup. He had a return station on the side, so seconds and thirds didn't require waiting in line. Amtrak held the 2013 Davis Phinney Foundation Ride the Rockies record at thirteen pancakes.

I was more into the smoothies. The smoothie makers would have anticipatory signs starting three miles out announcing their stands (and the next rest stop). Usually, we would arrive at the rest stop very thirsty with two empty water bottles; by the fourth one, I was buying them two at a time. I would create an efficient smoothie fountain, holding them so that one refilled as the other poured into my mouth. The copious Mountain Dews gave me a sugar and caffeine boost, but probably dehydrated me due to their diuretic effect.

We were supposed to have one more pass to climb, and then it looked to be mostly downhill for the final two days. Because I have a healthy sense of denial, I ignored the fact that the finish line had been placed at a mountaintop resort. The night of the fifth day, we learned that the course planners had added over thirty miles and four thousand feet of climbing to the following day in order to circumvent some forest fires. I was glad that we were still going to make it to Canon City, but I was now equally concerned about the ninety-four miles we had to ride to get there. How bad was Hardscrabble Pass?

I decided that I was going to have to ensure that my ducks were in a perfect row. Like playing a harp, each string would have to be tuned optimally. The variables of sleep, meds, DBS amplitude, nutrition, and hydration would have to be in perfect balance.

I felt my best for most of the day. I must not have looked as good as I felt, because I was asked if I was okay on no fewer than twenty separate occasions during the ride. Apparently, I was in a Bikram half-moon yoga pose to the left, which would understandably concern people. I was just happy to be feeling good; I was well beyond the point of always trying to look good, too. I was thankful for the concern of others, and once they saw the "Foundation for Parkinson's" line on my Davis Phinney Foundation jersey, they seemed to figure it out. The cycling spirits rewarded us with a nice descent from Hardscrabble.

That night, I stood up in front of the large group of cyclists and announced to the crowd, "I have Parkinson's disease, and I can't believe I've ridden every mile!" I wanted to give testament to what could still be done with proper motivation and support—and hopefully inspire others with Parkinson's to do what they could, too, even if it was just walking across the living room. I thanked the Davis Phinney Foundation for suggesting that I tackle Ride the Rockies, and also for the tremendous support they had provided. I also thanked everyone who had shown concern for me, and assured them I was all right. I ended by asking Dan to stand up so I could publicly convey my gratitude.

Anyone who is faced with a major illness or other life-changing events knows that you find out who your real friends are. These are people like my friend Willie, who came out to stay with me after my DBS surgery for a week, to make sure I was okay and provide comic relief. My wife, Cheryl, who didn't sign up for a husband with PD, but still loves me and supports me and is always there for me. Also, people like Dan, who showed incredible patience and support to get me through this ride and didn't hesitate when asked to do it. I realize now more than ever that I depend on others, and it is only more important that I appreciate it, and show them how thankful I am. I couldn't have ridden the Rockies without Dan.

Today we rode around a wildfire that unfortunately torched the Royal Gorge Bridge and surrounding buildings. The people of Canon

City are so nice and happy to have us here. So we rode ninety-four miles, with two major climbs and big descents. Afterward, I got up onstage and thanked my wingman Dan and the Davis Phinney Foundation. Thank you, too, for all of your support. I did it! Every mile plus.

I think my older daughter's letter to Dan after the ride said it best:

> I am completely amazed at and grateful for all that you did for my dad. Thank you so much for riding behind my dad and not passing him. That means a lot to me, because I know that sometimes it's hard to be patient and slow down, but you stayed with my dad no matter how tired he was, so you could watch out for him and be his friend. I was a little worried about my dad doing such a long ride, and I am so relieved to hear that he was never alone. Also, I think you deserve a very special badge of honor because, as I heard, you carried in my dad's luggage as well as your own when my dad was really tired. I cannot thank you enough. Also, I especially love hearing stories from the ride, because you can be really funny!

There were forty-four miles of cycling between me and the finish line. I celebrated crossing it with four Venti-sized Starbucks cups full of ice and Mountain Dew.

> Completed the ride today. Total miles for the week-five hundred and forty-six. I think the ride router had kind of a sick sense of humor, because he kept throwing steeper and steeper hills at us right to the end. They also announced

that this was the longest course in the twenty-six year history of Ride the Rockies. I'm now on the plane home. Can't wait to see my family!

STILL GOT IT

Doubt whom you will, but never yourself.
—Christian Nestell Bovee

I worked at a busy and rewarding center for cardiac surgery for thirteen years. The day I decided to retire was eight years after my diagnosis of Young-Onset Parkinson's disease, and four years after the implantation of my Deep Brain Stimulator. Up until the last day, I worked a full schedule. There was never, to my knowledge, a complaint from a patient or surgeon related to my Parkinson's disease.

In 1990, the Americans with Disabilities Act (ADA) was enacted. This meant that I had the right to reasonable workplace accommodations as long as I could otherwise do my job safely and effectively. Thank you, President Clinton.

I had recently been on the search committee for our new chairman, and his fairness was one of the reasons why I had endorsed him. He would have provided accommodations for me even without the development of ADA. My division director, and immediate boss, was equally accommodating.

Right after my diagnosis, I didn't need much in terms of workplace accommodation. I felt competent to do my job, but the accessibility was a welcome precaution. I positioned myself as residency director, which meant that I was responsible for making the residents' schedules and maintaining room assignments. I was therefore able to ensure that I was teaching a senior, experienced resident at all times, rather than a newer, lesser-experienced resident.

Of course, I had to be able to step in and place the lines or intubate when necessary, but training an experienced resident meant that I would have to do that less often, enabling me to maintain my dopamine stores.

With Parkinson's, we do make some dopamine; we just have less of it, and if we can conserve our movements and mental stress, we have more of a reserve for later. Eventually, I voluntarily stopped taking calls, and it was mandated that I never work alone. This was not only for patient safety, but also to protect myself, and it worked. I was able to safely and effectively work without problems.

Once my DBS was implanted, it added another level of safety and reserve to the mix. I would feel relatively comfortable and safe on no meds, with the DBS cranked up. I usually didn't tell the patients I had PD, although I'm sure it was fairly obvious to them. Just when I thought I was looking normal I would get a comment about my walk or get asked by a stranger if I was okay. I took very seriously, however, my responsibility as a professional to be able to perform my job and do it well. Moreover, as a senior anesthesiologist, I had to be one of the best, given my years of experience. In the back of my mind, I always knew that I would retire before I became a burden on anyone.

Over the course of my entire career, I probably performed ten thousand anesthetics. For each patient, however, it was usually his or her first time. To them, it wasn't just another day at the office, but a much bigger deal. The anesthetic wasn't first and foremost in their minds, though; it was something they may have taken entirely for granted. For them, the reason for the surgery represented the real focus; the anesthetic was just a necessary part of the day. If you asked most of my patients today who their anesthesiologist had been, they would surely have no idea. Most people just assume that the hospital will supply them with a competent person, and never give it a second thought.

With the onset of my neurological symptoms, it was my turn to become a patient. In the hospital, it's a bit like there are two teams. The medical staff is the one with the advantage; they are always on their home held, and they are usually healthy. They get to go home at the end of the day or walk away from the bedside and go have lunch with friends. What I understood from being a patient in the hospital was the disregard of the medical staff toward the reality of illness. Sure, they will help you and will take pride in doing so, but they won't be able to actually feel your pain, and they won't notice the way the illness has changed your life and that of your family. Even the most compassionate of doctors can't fully empathize with the devastation of being ill. I don't hold anyone at fault for that. It's human nature, a necessary condition that allows doctors and nurses to do their best work. Otherwise, the sorrow and anxiety associated with the profession would be overwhelming.

What I learned as a patient made me a better doctor. I now understand the experience from the sharp side of the needle. It's the little things, like the disorienting view of the ceiling on the way around the hospital. They don't allow you to walk, and keep you confined to a bed. With the advent of my own illness, my upside-down eyes immediately became more comforting to my patients as their last view of the world prior to surgery. I now know that a calm, confident voice is the most compassionate gift, the one patients truly need. They are usually not concerned with the details of the anesthetic.

My innate understanding of Parkinson's disease allowed me to help two patients in particular, and this was incredibly fulfilling. A woman in her eighties was having her aortic valve replaced through a needle stick—a transcatheter arterial aortic valve replacement. Most people—and by most, I mean almost everybody—would not have noticed her stillness, slow speech, soft, mumbled voice, and lack of movement. To the greater part of society, she looked like a typical eighty-year-old. I knew she had Parkinson's disease, which becomes even more common in the ninth decade of life, and therefore goes undiagnosed with greater frequency. Although it looks normal to us, it causes a lot of discomfort to the patient.

We finished the procedure, and as soon as she was able to follow a command to swallow, I gave her the medication. Several minutes later, we all watched as her eyes opened wider. It appeared that life had returned to her mind and body. To the staff in the room, it was as if I had performed a miracle. I hadn't. I just knew that she could feel better, move faster, and speak more clearly with a little dopamine. Usually, to us Parkies, transition from *off* to *on* happens in a highly acute manner, like flipping a switch. I always say that it feels so good, it's almost worth having the disease. Almost.

As DBS surgery becomes more common, an increasing number of patients come to surgery for other reasons with a DBS already in place. Most patients are uncomfortable turning it on and off, or even adjusting it themselves. We had a tongue cancer patient with DBS come to surgery twice in a two-month period. He and his family acted like I had the keys to their kingdom, because I was able to turn his DBS down, and off for his surgery; and more importantly, give him the ability to move after he woke up again.

It is so important to empower yourself with knowledge so that as a patient, you can have a major say in all aspects of your care. To date, being a patient is much like getting on an airplane. Like pilots, the doctors have most of the knowledge and control over your journey. There is one important difference, however. The pilots are in the planes with the passengers. That fact alone puts both pilots and passengers on the same team. The best way to get on the same team as the doctors who are treating you is to acquire as much knowledge as you can about your situation.

A new movement called "Patient Directed Care" does just that. The doctors become consultants, and the patients are given medical as well as nonmedical options, and choose their own destiny. This is extremely important with Parkinson's patients. We know best how we feel minute to minute, and therefore may make adjustments in the timing of our meds. We know which exercises make us feel better, and if we don't, it is so important that we find out. There don't have to be two different teams. Having been on both, I know how important it is that we unite as one toward a common goal.

A HOUSE FULL OF PARKIES

Whatever you vividly imagine, ardently desire, sincerely believe,
and enthusiastically act upon… must inevitably come to pass!
—Paul J. Meyer

It's amazing how quiet snowfall can be.

I was leaving a beautiful log cabin just below Peak 8 in
Breckenridge, Colorado, where I had been staying for a week with a
dozen others struggling with Parkinson's disease. As I walked down
the long, snow-covered walkway, the snow was quickly blanketing
everything I could see. It was as dark as it was silent and majestic. I
took a deep breath of the crisp, cool air at an elevation of ten thousand feet, and then reflected on how fulfilling the preceding week
had been. I was leaving in the predawn darkness for an airport shuttle
after an incredible week filled with laughter and tears, perspiration
and inspiration, and the sharing of our own personal experiences
with Parkinson's disease.

Breckenridge is home to the Breckenridge Outdoor Education
Center, which uses physical activity as experiential therapy for a myr-
iad of physical and psychological issues. I had been invited by a doctor from Oregon to their winter Parkinson's week. I had never met
him before, but through the miracle of YouTube—he was my only
follower—he had seen me ski. The doctor was volunteering as an
example of independent skiing with Parkinson's, and he wanted me
to join him and do the same.

I jumped at the chance to hang out and compare notes for a
week with other people impacted by Parkinson's. Two weeks before I
left for Breckenridge, I had mentioned the course to the CEO of the

Davis Phinney Foundation who was eager to put information about it on their website. The course filled up quickly, and when I arrived, every bed in the log cabin was filled either with a Parkie or a support buddy.

I noticed that most of the Parkies present had brought a family member or friend along for support, rather than travel alone. Those of us with Parkinson's disease covered a wide range of ages, and we were all differently affected. No two looked the same.

There was young Maureen who was only about forty years old and had never skied before. She had been recently diagnosed. Ironically, she was a physical therapist for movement disorders. As if Parkinson's were somehow contagious, she had been diagnosed as well. A woman named Diane, who was in her seventies, was a former ski instructor who hadn't been able to ski in ten years, and just wanted to have the experience of skiing with her granddaughter. She was my favorite, because she reminded me of my Grandma Bert who had Parkinson's disease in her seventies.

Two men, both named Roy, were the most inspiring. Although they had more severe symptoms, they loved to ski fast, and with the adaptive ski instructors, they were able to do so. One Roy had no voice and a very small, shuffling gait; but with an outrigger and a chest harness, he skied with incredible speed. The other Roy had serious postural problems; he was stuck forward and bent over, and therefore wheelchair-bound. He could travel forty miles per hour in a chair ski-harnessed to an adaptive ski instructor who trailed behind him.

There was something about living together that was liberating. We Parkies understood each other's struggles and issues beyond our control, such as snoring or screaming while asleep, for example. There also exists a phenomenon whereby merely being around others with PD can make some of our symptoms improve tremendously. Some people may begin to speak more clearly. I skied the best I ever had since my diagnosis. Some people conjecture that this occurs because we are not self-conscious, so there is less cortical input and more old ingrained memory guiding our actions. We skied only six hours a day, did yoga, and shared exercise and medication experiences with each other.

I had a soft spot for Diane, the seventy-one-year-old former ski instructor. I wanted to help her get her confidence back on skis so she could ski with her granddaughter. She had a fantastic adaptive instructor, and I just tagged along as her moral support. The first day, she was frozen stiff. I couldn't tell if it was from the PD or if she was simply terrified. On her first run in ten years, she lost control and ended up in the woods. The instructor took off quickly after her, and caught her before she fell. After that, that instructor held onto Diane closely for two days. Eventually, Diane told me to go explore the mountain, so I did.

Returning on day three, I found her skiing well, solo on greens and blues, and looking fully like an instructor again. Out of nowhere, and as the result of a lot of patience, Diane's confidence had magically returned. Her granddaughter would be so happy. She left for home at the end of that week with a big smile on her face. I had done nothing but shown her that Parkinson's doesn't mean you can't ski.

Maureen, the young Parkie, sent me a touching e-mail after we were all home:

> Jon,
>
> You were more of a help than you obviously know. It truly was a pleasure to meet you. I am grateful that you were there and thankful that you answered all of my many questions about DBS so patiently and thoroughly. More than anything you said, it was by observing you that I got to see the tangible benefit of surgery. You didn't need to stand up in front of the group and pontificate as others did. Your point was eloquently made by the way you carry yourself and by the evidence of the full life that you lead.
>
> I hope our paths will cross again.

Six months later, wonderful news!

Dear Jon,

I guess I've been remiss in telling you just how big of an impact you made on me but it's been a busy summer… In part, because of your example, on Wednesday, July 30th of this year, I underwent twelve hours of DBS surgery at the University of Arizona Medical Center. Four days later, I was out running errands, having come through the surgery better than anyone would have expected.

I was "programmed and activated" two weeks later when my doctors instructed me to stop taking my carbidopa/levodopa cold turkey. About two to three weeks after that I wound up back in the hospital for four days until they figured out that my 104 degree fever and stabbing headaches were caused by neuroleptic malignant-like syndrome. I spent the next two weeks in bed but have come through the crisis to be better than new! Even despite the complications, I would do it again every day of the week.

With my overall decline being so slow and insidious and my attitude of always trying to make lemonade from lemons, it is simply staggering how much of my life DBS has given back! It's as if someone has rolled back the clock by a dozen years!

Here is a partial but growing list of the newfound possibilities DBS surgery has brought:

1. Relieved tremor and stiffness
2. I'm (almost) medfree!
3. My right arm swings!
4. Ankle mobility

5. I can pet both of my dogs at the same time again!
6. I can cook again!
7. I can pursue my advanced kettlebell certification!
8. Washed my hair with both hands
9. Can apply makeup and brush teeth with right hand
10. I can write whenever I want
11. I can work with clients all day without having to stop and eat to take a pill
12. I can stretch clients without being embarrassed by a tremor
13. Poured and drank wine with my right hand and held the glass by only the stem!
14. I can run again only now nothing hurts.
15. I can type
16. Cross patterning isn't confusing anymore.
17. I'm very comfortable on the treadmill again. I don't list to right anymore and feel uncoordinated.
18. Increased RPM on my bike by a third from 60 to 90!

So it's been all great news until you consider the huge financial hit I took during all of that. I have absolutely no vacation time left and I probably won't be able to get away this year. It's a shame too because I would like to stand shoulder to shoulder with you as a DBS example.

I cannot thank you enough for attending last year. I hope you will continue to go in my absence.

Your friend,
Maureen

We are all in this together. Every Parkie in the world is on the same team. Sometimes, it just takes someone who understands what you are going through to make you feel better. It is most unsettling to be in a situation where no one knows you have Parkinson's, and therefore you can't do what they expect of you. Davis Phinney once said, "You tell someone you have PD, they join your team." Someone with PD is already there. Lessons from the Arctic tell me one plus one equals three. Just think about what a whole team can do.

BIG AND LOUD

Sometimes silence can be the loudest thing.
—Ellie Mathews

About once a year, the movement-disorder Fellows at the hospital change. They're neurologists, gaining extra diagnostic experience, and treating disorders such as Parkinson's, dystonia, Tourette's, restless leg syndrome, essential tremor, chorea… the list goes on. By far, the most common is Parkinson's. On my semiannual visits, they will usually see me first, and then my attending neurologist will agree or disagree with their assessment and plan. It's nice to meet new Fellows, because they're creative. They're too young to be set in their ways, and are always looking for new ways to help me.

Last year, my new Fellow wanted to know if I had ever been offered LSVT (Lee Silverman Voice Training) BIG and LOUD therapy. Before that day, I had never heard of it. It is designed specifically for Parkinson's patients, because we tend to make small, careful movements and speak softly. This just gets worse if we make no attempts to counteract it.

I called the physical therapy department to schedule my appointment, and found out that you have to do BIG therapy first. The scheduler said, "We always do BIG first. You don't want to be small and loud, do you? Let's make you big, and then we will get you loud!"

BIG is a series of repetitive large movements in an attempt to remodel the brain, and make larger motions more natural. Led by a specifically trained physical therapist, these exercises are done an hour a day, four times a day, for four weeks. At first, the motions can be difficult and frustrating, but by the end of the four weeks, they feel much more natural. The benefits are maintained by doing the exercises daily on your own. In an attempt to make your voice louder, the therapist also has you count very loudly to keep track of how many times you have repeated a motion. However, this is not LOUD therapy.

LOUD is done with a speech pathologist. The goal is to strengthen your vocal cords and muscles of speech by having you repeatedly hold a loud tone for as long as you can. My record was thirty-seven seconds. I showed up four days a week for four weeks, and graduated from the program with honors! I found the big movements exhilarating, and it was also fun to measure how I was speaking—then make it louder. At one point, the therapist told me I was being too loud!

Afterward, I wanted to find a way to continue the BIG exercises, while making them less monotonous and more enjoyable. I saw an ad on TV for the New York Trapeze School, and for about a day, I was planning to do that. I partook in a session at the trapeze school, amazing my family because I was able to swing on the trapeze and hang from my knees. However, the repeated falling onto the net caused a black-and-blue mark over my generator. Fun as it was, I determined that I wanted an activity that would force me to make big, challenging movements, and give me agility, flexibility, and strength without the bruising.

Ultimately, I found exactly what I was looking for in rock climbing. It seemed a little safer and less traumatic to my DBS and wires.

I called around, and eventually found a private instructor who would let me climb in the morning when I could have the whole gym to myself. I showed up the first day, and found out that the only criterion to climb was to possess a fearlessness of heights.

I learned that walls are all different; some angled in, others angled out. A few have an overhang. They are all rated by the route setter. The first number, five, means you don't need anything but a belay rope to climb it. The easiest climb in the gym is a 5.5, and they become progressively harder, all the way up to 5.13. The major factors with climbing include making large movements to reach and grab for holds with all four limbs. It also involves strengthening core muscles to stabilize yourself on the wall. Most importantly, it's very challenging for the thinking part of your brain. Like a constant puzzle, while climbing, you are figuring out the route in order to be most balanced and save energy.

On my first day, I attempted a 5.6 and could make it only halfway up. Over the course of a year, I have progressed to the point where I can reliably climb a 5.7 without falling, and complete many 5.8s as well. Certain climbs really test my tenacity. I spent a full forty minutes on one particular 5.8, and while attempting a big move in the middle, I fell approximately twenty times. I refused to come down. Eventually, I dug down deep inside, made the maximum possible effort, and ascended to the top. That particular climb actually became easier and easier as the weeks passed. Usually, I feel great on the wall. I don't know if it's the stretching or sense of accomplishment or both.

In rock climbing, it's a person versus gravity. That's all there is to it. The holds are in set locations on the wall, and once you choose your path, it cannot change. You can only alter your technique to make it easier in the moment or you can wait until you naturally get stronger just from repeated attempts to climb a difficult wall. I have definitely become more flexible with increased muscle mass and strength during the first year. This, along with more efficient form and improved balance, has led to my progression up the "five" scale. I have a long way to go.

I felt so much immediate and long-term benefits from rock climbing that I started a group climb once a week. My LSVT BIG physical therapist came out to climb with us, and she agreed about the benefits in relation to Parkinson's symptoms. We wrote an article together for the Georgetown University Hospital Movement Disorders Newsletter. She has also been sending her BIG graduates to me, and our Wednesday climbing group is rapidly growing and creating rock climbing addicts. We all feel better on the wall.

It has been two years now, and what is most important to me is that I always finish a climb once I've started it, no matter how many times I fall. The climbing center is where somebody first called me tenacious after I spent forty minutes getting up a difficult climb. I think I can beat Parkinson's with tenacity. I may move slower, but if I keep turning over the pedals, taking another step under that canoe or attempting to climb, eventually I will succeed.

THE HOT ROOM

Do you know a cure for me? Salt water in one way
or the other. Sweat, tears or the salt sea."
—Isak Dinesen

One Sunday, in the middle of winter, I was invited by Juice to an introductory yoga class. I didn't know that it was going to be hot yoga or that it was ninety minutes long. Before I knew it, I was standing next to Juice, trying my best to balance on one leg with sweat pouring off my body like an open kitchen faucet. This would have been hard enough at seventy-two degrees. After thirty minutes at one hundred five degrees, I thought I was going to pass out. I tried to follow the instructor's simple instructions. "Whatever you do, don't leave the room."

The thing about hot yoga is that, for some reason, about two hours after the class, a feeling of invigoration spreads throughout the body. It's more than just the stretching. Two mornings a week, I spend ninety minutes attempting the same twenty-six poses in a pool of sweat. Yoga forces me to open joints and stretch muscles that have become very tight over many years. We individuals with Parkinson's tend to be in a vicious cycle; we move less because we are tight, and we are tighter because we move less. I am determined to break that cycle.

The thing I like about Bikram Yoga is that it's the same twenty-six poses in the same order every time. I can go to Bikram Yoga anywhere and know what to expect. Even if I am in a foreign country, and don't speak the language, I can practice, because I have done the poses so many times exactly the same way.

I am always the worst in the class. The instructors make it look so effortless.

After one of my initial classes, I said to the instructor, "I have a long way to go!"

She replied, "We all have a long way to go."

What a great philosophy for life. I will never stop learning, giving, improving, trying, failing, and trying again. Even the instructor can improve and get more out of her yoga practice.

I've often wondered why the room needed to be so hot. The teachers will tell you that they keep it hot because you sweat out the toxins or that your muscles and joints will stretch better. The best explanation I heard was from ChauKei Ngai, the woman's international Bikram Yoga champion who came to visit us, teach a class, and give a demonstration. She said they keep it hot to teach you to stay calm and focused, and ignore adversity. She even tells you not to wipe your sweat with a towel, just look past it.

I have often been asked if I feel self-conscious being half-naked in a room doing yoga poses, making it obvious that I have Parkinson's disease. The answer is no. I have nothing to hide. I didn't choose to have Parkinson's, and I have found it liberating to tell people I have it. They become part of my team. People are generally very supportive, and once they know, I am no longer clumsy, slow, and awkward. For some reason, I become "inspiring."

Parkinson's would like to make me stiff, tight, quiet, and small. No way was I going to let that conquer me! A person has to fight back. They can attack it with exercise, with stretching, with yoga, with rock climbing. The person "ailing" from Parkinson's disease should make sure to stay in the game, socialize, and speak to people. The more one does for himself or herself, the more they can do and the more they will do.

I always tell people with Parkinson's to ignore the heat. Invite people to join their team. Tell them about the struggle with Parkinson's disease, even about its little nuances. If a person does so, they will soon discover that everyone has a struggle of some sort. You can help them as much as they can help you.

We all have a long way to go.

The most intelligent thing I have ever heard about free advice is that you get what you pay for. We all have a different experience on this Earth. We may think we have a solid plan, but the only absolute truth is that nothing is absolute. Having your life plan altered could be compared to jumping off a cliff; we will eventually land, and hopefully, softly. We never know exactly where we'll come down, though, and this can create a significant source of anxiety.

First of all, empower yourself by getting organized. In my case, I felt as if I had lost complete control of my body, and it therefore became imperative to have all other aspects of my life in complete control. I met with a financial planner, and made sure I had jumped through all of the appropriate hoops for my disability insurance. Then I focused exclusively upon my physical and mental health.

Exercise, in and of itself, is both beneficial and monumentally important for people with Parkinson's disease. This is a disease of rest, not intention. It tends to want to lock you into a stiff, unbalanced prison, but with the proper motivation, you can actually break the chains of Parkinson's disease. The more you move, the more you can move. I believe it is important to exercise your mind, as well. Learn something new. Do puzzles. Help others.

I have found such immense benefit in the daily exercises I do involving BIG movements, balance, and agility. A basic law of physics says that things at rest tend to stay at rest, while things in motion tend to stay in motion. What actually consumes our energy is initiating and stopping movements, or changing direction. Neuroplasticity is a fancy word for the ability to intentionally relearn how to accelerate, decelerate, and change direction quickly. We can remodel our brains; we just have to challenge them. The more we move, the more we can move. It seems simple, but it's true.

MEETING THE CHALLENGE

May you live all the days of your life.
—Jonathan Swift

Fourteen miles north of Washington, DC, roars Great Falls, a gorgeous but treacherous section of the Potomac River. Deceitfully, the strong currents and powerful waterfalls are just out of view, making the eddy pools that you do see look inviting on a hot summer day. Since my early childhood, I recall the impressive sign by the overlook to the falls, which was updated annually with the number of deaths per year from people swimming or falling into that section of the Potomac River. Just below the falls are rapids suitable for kayaking and rock faces great for climbers who have the skill and gear.

I knew about the Billy Goat Trail, a hiking trail between the canal and the Potomac, but I guess I had never really been on it. I may have been on sections B or C as a kid; they are shorter and less difficult than A, because what I was picturing in my mind—when I recommended that we hike the trail for Julie's birthday—was a nice leisurely hike through the woods. Julie and I even brought a picnic lunch to eat halfway through while enjoying the view.

The morning of Julie's nineteenth birthday was overcast and drizzly with the promise of afternoon thunderstorms. We decided to go on the hike anyway; the weather would be actually very comfortable, and we brought puzzles to do in the car if the storms came. We walked the mile and a half on the towpath to the Billy Goat Trail entrance. Of course, I stopped at the famous warning sign to show Julie about the danger of the Falls. What I didn't see was the plain as day caution sign at the entrance to the trail.

This posting in big bold letters basically said that there are three Billy Goat Trails and that we were on A, the most challenging of the three. It said the hiker must be a "physically fit adult" to "attempt" this trail. Parts of it are slippery and treacherous. It advised us to wear sticky-soled shoes and bring plenty of water, because it would probably require three hours. It follows the Potomac River Gorge, so if you fall in the water, it will be difficult to get out. I might have channeled Arctic Trip Fred and taken the smart road if I had read that sign before we entered the trail.

Luckily, we had plenty of water and rubber-soled shoes. The first hour of walking was challenging, but doable, even for a guy with a movement disorder. We let some people go by, but I erroneously thought the whole walk would take about an hour. Then came the sign. In big bold letters, it warned us that the trail got much more difficult for the two hours left, with steep climbing and jumps. In my mind it said, "If you have Parkinson's disease, turn around or you will get hurt!"

I was really considering going back, taking the safe choice. A man came by with his two daughters. "I have done it a million times; you will be fine!"

I had, of course, to take into consideration that he didn't know I had PD. So along came two Physical Therapy students. I knew they had some medical knowledge, because they were talking about neurologic disorders. This was my chance. If I told them I had PD, then I would have that much more support for the rest of the hike. Sure, Julie is the best, and very supportive, but she is also my daughter, my responsibility. This is one of those times that telling someone you have PD changes you in their eyes from clumsy to an inspiration. So since we had water, new friends, two charged cell phones and clearing weather, I decided to go for it carefully, knowing we always had plenty of time to turn back.

If I hadn't had two years of indoor rock-climbing under my belt, I would have been in trouble. What I lacked in balance and proprioception, I had to make up for by using my hands all the time— grabbing trees, roots, vines, rocks, and even crawling when I had no other choice. The dark gray moss covered jagged edges of rock pointed straight to the bluing sky. Those with balance would stand tall and walk across them as if crossing a balance beam. I didn't trust my balance at first, so I would use all four extremities so as not to fall into the small crevices between the rocks. Twenty minutes into that section, I was holding onto the steep rock, sweat pouring from my forehead, and wondering if I had made the right choice. Julie was easily navigating, so I asked her if she could carry the backpack. Of course she could! "No problem, Dad!"

Taking off the backpack, my glasses, and my watch gave me freedom. As time went on, my brain adapted to the situation. My balance improved and I picked up speed. Every ten minutes or so, someone would easily coast by me, reminding me I have an impairment.

Before we knew it, we were at the third sign. Even though the wording was about the same, inside my head the message was different: "You've done the hardest part, it won't get any harder or they would tell you."

We passed the midpoint emergency exit. By now, I had embraced the struggle. We were following light blue paint on the rocks, which showed us the way. We learned to trust the blue paint even when it led us over small mountains of rock. On the way down those rock faces, I would always find a good handhold or tree or strong vine for support. During this last hour, to our right was the beautiful Potomac River Gorge, which had sheer cliffs on either side. An hour later, we had climbed out of there and were back on the towpath having lunch.

Parkinson's is a dynamic process. If you let it win, it will. If you challenge it, you will be pleasantly surprised. At the same time, I felt that we were always safe. We enlisted support and always had a Plan B.

FIRST RESPONDER

There is no exercise better for the heart than
reaching down and lifting people up.

—John Holmes

I sat glued to the television, watching John Gage and Roy DeSoto arrive on the scene to rescue someone who had choked on a pop-top. As a child, I was always fascinated by those brave enough to try to help in a medical emergency. If asked back then what I wanted to be, I would have said that I wanted to become a banker; however, I must have inherited the medical gene. I always wanted to have the knowledge base to be able to provide aide as a First Responder. Although I took the Red Cross Advanced First Aid course in high school, and again in college, I felt most comfortable in emergency situations after I became a doctor. On the other hand, I can become frustrated by limitations of being without the proper medications or equipment when faced with an out-of-hospital situation.

Halfway across the Atlantic Ocean, on an Air France flight to Paris, I heard an announcement in French, which I didn't understand.

"It sounds like they're looking for a doctor," the person beside me said.

I leaned into the aisle and looked back to see a large blue man sitting in the last row. As I hurried to him, many thoughts rushed through my mind. I tried to think of all the reasons to turn blue on an airplane, most of which are cured by oxygen. He was breathing and audibly wheezing when I got there. Luckily, his English-speaking friend told me his history. He had asthma and had gotten on the plane standby without his inhaler. Just removing him from his seat and freeing up his shirt seemed to help. I asked for oxygen, expecting it to fall from above; instead, they brought me an oxygen canister and a box of French medications. I didn't recognize the French inhaler, but luckily our patient did.

As he turned pink again and felt better, the flight attendant asked me if there was anything else I needed.

I jokingly replied, "How 'bout a seat in first class?"

Not knowing I was joking, she said, "What a great idea!"

She then brought our asthma victim to first class.

I was glad. He needed it more than I did.

Another time, although she faints at the thought of blood, my daughter Julie remained very calm and called for help twice while I was assisting two others who had become injured. The first incident happened in National Airport. We were returning from a family ski trip. Julie and I were headed to the parking lot to get the car when I saw a woman lying flat on the ground at the end of a moving walkway, and people stepping over her to get past. I saw from afar that she was convulsing and told Julie to call 911 while I ran to her. Without oxygen or suction, all I could do was open her airway to let her breathe. Her breath smelled like acetone as she began to awaken from the pain from the jaw thrust I was giving to her.

I said to her, "You're either diabetic, epileptic or drunk."

She smiled and said, "That would be the latter!"

A TSA officer who was close arrived. I waited for the ambulance to come, and then Julie and I were on our way.

The second time, Julie was riding her bike behind me one day on the Capitol Crescent Trail near our home when we were first on the scene after a bike versus pedestrian crash, which we didn't see. I knew this, because I saw two victims lying on the ground, each in a pool of their own blood, and only one bike. They were both awakening, and the bleeding had stopped. There wasn't much to do but ask them not to move until the rescue squad arrived. Although I was worried, it turned out that Julie doesn't faint at the sight of other peoples' blood. She had remained calm and called for help. Great job, Julie!

Of course, my most memorable event involved me as the victim. I had to save my own life. I was in medical school having lunch with two friends, Vera and Randy, at the Penn restaurant behind the University of Maryland medical school. I had eaten there many times before. These were two of my closest group of friends in medical school, and we were always telling jokes.

As the three of us were laughing, I inhaled a large piece of mozzarella cheese, and soon they were giggling alone. I couldn't move air in or out of my lungs. Time slowed down. My first thought was to use the Levine sign, the international sign for choking; then one of them would Heimlich me by thrusting their fists up under my rib cage and dislodging the cheese. I was in a room full of hospital personnel—surely someone would save me.

None of this happened. Vera and Randy were laughing and telling jokes as I sat, silently dying. Time began to speed up. I had to get some air. I don't know where I learned it, but it was in my repertoire. I knew how to do the Heimlich maneuver on myself. I dove across the table, landed on my fists, and coughed up the cheese. I reached into my throat, and grabbed the bolus, and pulled it the rest of the way out. I knocked plates, glasses, and silverware off the table in a loud commotion. My friends just looked at me as if to say, "Why didn't you say something?"

Helping someone "in the held" often required some imagination. Assisting these patients was bound to be outside my comfort zone—certainly, the environment would differ from my usual routine. I had to have the confidence that I most likely had the knowledge to help. The only way to find out was to try. I realized the older and wiser I became, it was important to recognize that which I didn't know—the least I can do is show up.

WHEN FAMILY CALLS

Other things may change us, but we start and end with family.
—Anthony Brandt

I am incredibly grateful that I engaged in a career as a cardiac anesthesiologist. After years of working with heart attack patients, I had learned very well how to recognize and treat the life-threatening situation known as acute myocardial infarction or MI. My knowledge had not been attained just for my patients. Should a friend or family member ever find him or herself in need, I felt confident that I had made the necessary connections over the course of my career to treat them. I had the crucial phone numbers programmed into my phone to access the proper channels and stop an MI in its tracks. As we say in the business, "time is heart muscle." It helps to know the system.

It must have been late summer, because I remember I had just returned from the beach wearing a torn T-shirt and sandals, and my shorts were full of sand. I received a terrifying call. Scott, my little sisters husband, had collapsed while painting his bathroom, clutching his chest. I knew that he had super high cholesterol, because he had mentioned his cholesterol level at a family dinner a few months earlier. I also knew that the risk factors favored an MI, and that was the only life-threatening diagnosis that fit the symptoms.

By the time I arrived at their house, I had to insist that the ambulance take Scott to the nearest hospital. The EMTs thought it was only a panic attack. Scott had the classic severe crushing chest pain, and first and foremost on my shortlist of possibilities was an MI. I followed the ambulance closely, and at one point on the way to the hospital, they pulled over to tell me that I should be running the red lights to follow them. It was all I could do to stay calm. I let them know to treat him like a heart attack victim, and ask questions later.

Although Scott had the classic symptoms and risk factor for a life-threatening MI, his EKG was not yet showing it; and therefore, even the doctors in the ER thought he just had indigestion. After waiting for a few minutes, I insisted that they let me into the ER. When I walked in, one of the doctors was asking Scott lots of questions and writing his history in the chart. I knew we had to act quicker than that. As the minutes ticked by, Scott was losing valuable heart muscle. I talked to Scott, and he said the discomfort was almost unbearable.

As I picked up the phone to talk to the cardiac surgeon on call, and began the chain of events that assembled the cardiac cath (cardiac catheterization) lab staff and the cardiac surgery team at our hospital, the EKG rhythm strip began to show the MI. It was worse than I feared; the EKG showed that the blockage was in the most major artery. Time was of the essence, so I also asked for the MedStar life flight chopper. I knew that keeping Scott calm was important. I tried to use that calm voice that airline pilots use during scary turbulence. I told him that it was his heart, but we knew what was wrong and how to fix it. I was transferring him to my hospital.

Like a scene from a movie, the backdoors to the helipad soon opened. Wind was blowing papers off tables and through the bays.

Scott asked, "What's that?"

I said, "That's your ride!"

After only four minutes of time in the air, he was at our hospital, and we went straight to our twenty-four-hour cath lab. The cardiologist put in a balloon pump, which is a device that forces blood past the blockages in coronary arteries. It's known to stop the MI right in its tracks. This was my everyday experience, but to this lawyer, who couldn't stand the sight of blood, it must have been a terrifying experience.

How do I know that Scott couldn't stand the sight of blood? Earlier that year, we were all visiting my parents at their cabin. My sister was at the kitchen sink, and had sliced a deep cut into her hand.

Having witnessed it, I said to Tina, "Are you okay?"

From behind me, collapsed on the couch, I heard Scott's voice, "I will be!"

So when the nurse removed the balloon pump later that day, and Scott got to see his own blood squirt up to the ceiling, he decided for sure that he had made the right choice: law school instead of medical school. Later, he would tell me that he didn't want to visit me at work ever again.

Thirty days and four surgeries later, including a bypass, Scott went home as healthy as ever. Of course, he did try to scare us one more time when he decided to sleep for two-and-a-half days post-op. As it turned out, he was just tired and needed a nap!

There were many days in my career that stood out, but the day of Scott's heart attack, I don't think I could have been more grateful that I attended medical school. I wasn't the treating doctor, but I had been able to expedite proper care of my relative because of my knowledge, experience, and connections.

This wasn't the first time I had put my training to use for my little sister's family. As a matter of fact, just six months earlier and five days after the birth of her second daughter, Johanna, she told me that the pediatrician had heard a heart murmur. She had gotten an ultrasound of her heart, and there was something wrong. The heart did have the normal four chambers, but there was some flow in the wrong direction in the mitral valve and some shunting of blood between the two sides of the heart. Normally, blood should all flow in a forward direction, not mix between the two sides. This was a tricky situation, because this baby had just been born, and while her heart was the size of a healthy plum, the mitral valve was only dime-sized.

I had always thought that fetal cardiac physiology and the transition at birth was very cool. Before a baby is born, it receives all of its oxygen through the umbilical vein coming from the mother. This oxygen-rich blood bypasses the lungs by passing across a hole between the two sides of the heart. This is supposed to close as the baby takes her first breath in response to the decrease in pressure in the right side of the heart. Like a door slamming shut, it should remain closed. However, in Johanna's case, it was clear that the door wasn't the right size to close the hole.

Although I had been trained in echocardiography, I knew I would need to call on the experts to help me evaluate this newborn's echo and guide my sister to the right doctors for her baby. I knew it was important not only to make the correct diagnosis, but also to know the natural history of the disease, which would tell us if and when to operate versus treating the condition with medication. Luckily, I worked on adult mitral valve cases for many years with an excellent mitral echocardiographer. She not only reviewed the echo, but she walked me next door to the children's hospital and got Johanna under the care of the right cardiologist and surgeon for her needs. Nine months later, she had surgery. She is now a thriving preteen with a surgical scar matching her dad's.

WINGS

Don't act your age in retirement. Act like the
inner young person you have always been.

—J. A. West

The day I decided to retire was like any other day. I drove to work that day at 5:30 a.m., as usual, and met my first patient at 6:00 a.m. It was June 4, 2012, the beginning of the month, and all the residents were new. I was working with one of my favorite surgeons. About 7:30 a.m., my meds started to wear off, and I began to slow down. This had happened before, but this time, my inner voice asked me, "How long are you gonna keep doin' this?" I called my partner to take over, and decided that it was the right day to go to full disability. All patients deserve a neuro-intact anesthesiologist.

Actually, it was like jumping off a cliff. I didn't know where I would land, but I knew for sure there was no going back. Should I have discussed it with Cheryl first? How much of my identity was tied to being a doctor? Thinking back, I retired at the right time.

Upon my retirement, it became difficult to face the fact that all of a sudden, I was no longer in the practice of medicine. After years and years of training and experience, I was out of the game. One of the best pieces of advice I received from my chairman was to take advantage of the time I now had, and do something I had always wanted to do if I only had the time.

I decided to learn to fly.

The Navy doctors who came through our program were usually older than the average resident, and often on their second career path. We had Marines, flight surgeons, pilots, submarine captains, etc. I would usually ask the pilots if they had a call sign, and most of them did, but not like in the movie Top Gun. The call signs were never cool, like "Maverick" or "Viper," but had been bestowed upon them during the initial training stages, and were therefore pseudo-derogatory in nature, like "G-spot," "Princess," and "Special Kay."

David "Special Kay" spent his four years of payback duty as the only anesthesiologist at the Cherry Point Naval Hospital. He had been an F-14 pilot in his first life, and now owned a small four-seater plane that he used to commute between Cherry Point, landing in New Bern, North Carolina, and his home in Norfolk, Virginia.

Once a year, in August, I would visit David on my way to pick up my daughter from summer camp with secret hopes of going flying. With this in mind, as we walked into a restaurant for dinner the August immediately following my retirement, I looked up at the blue sky and said, "Looks like a great night for flying!" It worked! He took the bait and offered us a tour of the Arapahoe Sound from the sky. I hadn't yet been trained in flight planning, so I didn't notice the sunset, and we were less than an hour away from nightfall.

After dinner, we headed over to the airport to find David's four-seater Mooney, gassed up and ready to go. We did a preflight check and actually kicked the tires. As we ascended to a low flying altitude, I felt a freedom from Parkinson's similar to what I normally felt on the bicycle. I was buckled in, and the plane was doing all the work. David was doing all of the necessary thinking, and after he offered me the controls, I was doing all the flying. I was "on the con," as they say, for the better side of an hour. I was able to ascend and descend, bank right and left, and even accomplish a sixty-degree turn that pulled about two Gs.

Darkness soon set in, and flying at night required the level of talent and experience David had. He said, "My aircraft;" and I said back, "Your aircraft," lifting my hands and feet from the controls. With many thousands of hours in the air, flying at night came naturally to David. He was able to land that plane as fast as he could set his F-14 onto the deck of an aircraft carrier. I guess it's comparable to the way I know how to manage an anesthetic after years of doing just that.

My first flight was incredibly uplifting, and purely enjoyable. For that hour, I was free of Parkinson's. Naturally, I wanted to do it again.

It just so happened that my good friend Dan, a.k.a. Amtrak, was getting back into flying. He had a license to fly small single-prop planes, and could fly VFR or by visual flight rules. I had flown with him once or twice twenty years earlier when we were roommates in medical school. Back then, we flew out of Baltimore Washington International Airport in line with commercial jets for takeoff and landing. It felt surreal to look to my left and see my buddy Dan about to take us to eight thousand feet. At that time, he was flying with the Dream Flight School out of Westminster, Maryland, in order to get his instrument rating.

I really thought that learning to fly was a crazy notion. Sure, I'd always wanted to learn, but I have Parkinson's disease! My balance and proprioception are off, my reflexes are slow, and I have no fine motor control. My ability to move depends upon a battery. If I did learn to fly, I would never get medical clearance to obtain a license, so I would never be able to fly alone. The cards were stacked against me, but I had to try. Understanding all of this, I signed up for a discovery flight to meet Jeremy, my instructor.

Jeremy somehow understood my need for flight and freedom from the things weighing me down on Earth. He agreed to teach me to fly as long as I always had a "safety pilot." For three months, I was a regular student. I learned take-off and did seven of them. I also did three landings, but I never got the feel of how to do it correctly. I would easily overshoot or undershoot, and Jeremy would verbally correct me. I could have used his voice in my ear years earlier, back when I was trying to catch fly balls!

I am glad I learned the basics of flight. It had been on my list of things I had always wanted to do. Even though it's called a bucket list, I don't plan to kick the bucket for a long time, so let's just call it my *wings* list. I'd had my wings clipped, so this was my "What I Now Get to See" list:

1. Learn to fly (check; done)
2. Bike through Europe (check; done)

3. Play the stock market (check; done)
4. Solve the Rubik's Cube (check; done)
5. Visit Australia (check; done)
6. Yoga (check; done)
7. Rock climbing (check; done)
8. Cycle the Rockies (check; done)
9. Meet Davis Phinney (check; done)
10. Meet Michael J. Fox (not yet)

Most people say this doesn't look like a list of someone with PD, but it does to me! I probably would have done most of these things if I didn't have Parkinson's. Am I just trying to prove to myself that I can do it? Is tenacity created through adversity?

As you can see, I am a very lucky man. I am truly blessed, and incredibly thankful for my family who give me my wings every day. Sure, Parkinson's forced me to retire early, but I now savor my many blessings rather than wallow in sorrow. I am able to spend a far greater amount of time with my wife and daughters. My *wings* list is mostly accomplished, and thanks to Medtronic, the Davis Phinney Foundation, my neurologist, and my neurosurgeon, I am able to help educate patients, caregivers, and medical staff so that they can best assist other Parkies in ending relief through DBS.-0

PERSEVERANCE—PART 4

The wilderness holds answers to questions
man has not yet learned to ask.
—Nancy Wynne Newhall

We were in true Canadian wilderness, a land untouched by the human race. It was as beautiful as God meant it to be. Our goal was to travel silently in our canoes, and leave minimal evidence of our passing. We didn't want to disturb the untamed splendor of this land. We would even practice what was known as "wet foot tripping," which meant we would hop out of our canoes before landing them on the shore in order to avoid destroying the shoreline with our canoes.

Surrounding us was a community of wildlife. The more we blended in with the pristine surroundings, the more we increased our chance of enriching our experience with the sighting of these magnificent creatures. We would see the loons daily. These expert fishermen birds are named for the sound they make, and unlike ducks, loons float just under the water with only their head above the surface. They have adapted to being less buoyant so they can more rapidly dive toward a school of fish. They wear a white stripe like a choker that sits at water level, reflecting light in such a way that they are less visible to their prey.

The deer in Canada come in three sizes. The white-tailed deer are the smallest of the three and are more prevalent in southern

Canada. The farther north you go, the more you will find the white-tail's larger cousin, the caribou. Bigger yet is Bambi's largest relative, the moose. Moose are huge. The adults weigh over a thousand pounds, and although they look cute, they are fierce. They have been known to attack humans who get too close, corner them or inadvertently come between parent and calf.

One evening, as we approached the shore to make camp, we saw an adult female moose swimming across the lake with her two calves right behind her. It had been a hard day of paddling, and it was such a beautiful vision to see the moose silhouette in the sun's rays coming through the trees. It was God's reward after such a trying day. As we reached the shore, it started to rain, which meant that I would be called upon that night for my special skill—starting a fire in the rain.

I would set out in search of birch trees, preferably fallen ones because, as Rory had taught me, birch bark will light even when wet. As I got farther from our campsite, I started to worry about that moose and her calves; I didn't want to get between them.

Vivid in my memory is what happened next. As I picked up a fallen birch log, I encountered a moose head. Not knowing at the time that this was the mostly skeletal remains of a moose—probably killed by its only predator, the polar bear—I turned and ran, startled, back to the campsite. Rory was excited. He had wanted a moose skull and rack to bring home, and commemorate his wilderness experience. We went back to retrieve it, and yes, there was a large set of antlers on it.

Rory spent every free minute of the next ten days carving the flesh off that skull. Also, Rory had a special place in his canoe for this thing, and he carried it on portages. I never really understood why he wanted it. It attracted insects, and my thought was that it might probably also attract bears. Rory had the same thought, because he hung it high in a tree every night with the food pack to keep from attracting bears to our tent sites.

It was more that I felt that we were in God's pure Canadian wilderness, and this was one of his beautiful creatures. It didn't really fit with our minimal impact ideals to remove that moose rack from this land. Later, I would find out that we all felt this way. Even Rory was conflicted.

Why didn't we say anything? Three weeks later, we would find out that things have a tendency to work out for the best.

It was a Class III rapids. We were days away from the end of our trip, and we were most likely overconfident in our ability to navigate whitewater. Class III is the highest level passable by a two-man canoe. usually, we would portage our gear around and paddle the empty canoes through the rapids with full spray skirts on. I don't know why, but Rory and I ended up on this challenge with a full canoe, including his moose rack—the spray skirt could only cover the bow and go around my waist. The second problem was that we couldn't see all of the rapids and had planned to "eddy out" halfway through and scout the rest. Eddies are areas behind large rocks where the water actually flows upstream, creating a calm space to stop and rest or regroup.

It is said that it usually takes three problems to create a disaster. Here came problem number three. As we spun around to eddy out, we missed the eddy and ended up traveling rapidly backward with the back of the canoe, with a spray skirt, taking on water. Next thing I knew, I was in the ice-cold North Seal River trying to stay calm and do what I had to do to survive, keeping my boots downstream, hitting rocks, and spinning around—it was all I could do to get my feet in front of me. I knew to get behind the boat and hold on to a line tied to the stern just for this reason.

Making it to shore, we took inventory. We had our packs and the canoe. The personal pack with clothes and sleeping bags had opened slightly, because the moose head was tied to it. The whitewater had claimed Rory's three weeks of work. The moose rack was gone! It was like God had taken it back to be forever in this piece of wilderness.

As important it was for me to return that skull and rack to the wilderness, I was more impressed by the relief we all talked about that the animal stayed where he belonged. Since then, I have learned to speak my mind more when something just doesn't feel right. That magnificent creature lived for many years in this pure land, and we all knew that it was best to leave him here. As we sat around the fire that night, wearing our soaking wet clothes in an effort to dry them out, we all confessed a hidden desire to leave the moose rack behind. Even Rory said it was for the best.

When I think back to my youth, my tenacious nature came about during this Arctic canoe trip. My successes showed me the importance of perseverance. I use this quality daily when fighting Parkinson's disease. At the same time, I know that we need to be safe, and moreover, considerate of all living creatures with whom we share this Earth. Tenacity can be beneficial but only when combined with the values of safety, health, and most importantly, *love*.

WHAT'S REALLY IMPORTANT

Don't sweat the small stuff... and it's all small stuff.
—Richard Carlson, PhD

Dealing with Parkinson's disease has taught me to appreciate what's really important in life. We share this Earth with over seven billion people, and I think we all find positive human interaction to be the most important thing. It's so easy to get caught up in the consumer phase of life, competing for the most respected profession, and the best schools for your kids, the big house, and a nice car. Everybody is trying to get their piece of the pie—and making it a big one. We are taught early on by society that this is the key to happiness. None of these things, however, correlates with real fulfillment. Helping people smile or get relief from seemingly insurmountable struggles is why we are actually here. The happiest people are those with the most love in their lives. Luckily, Parkinson's disease is not contagious, but a smile is.

Since my retirement, I have been so lucky to be able to spend more time with my amazing, beautiful wife and daughters. I can honestly say that I am truly happy when we are all together, laughing around the dinner table. Recently, I have found joy in helping others who struggle with Parkinson's. Sure, it significantly changes my life, but not necessarily for the worse. It's just different. It is still possible to live well with Parkinson's, and I intend to spread the word. I started the Parkinson's rock-climbing group because I want to show people that you can make big, strong movements, and it's amazing how good it feels. I will do the same for skiers with Parkinson's.

Since my diagnosis with Parkinson's, I have come to appreciate my family so much more. I have found my true friends and learned to make a difference through positive human interaction. This is the root of true happiness. It's the foundation of being me.

MEETING MY MENTOR

Tell me and I forget. Teach me and I
remember. Involve me and I learn.
—Benjamin Franklin

Jaws dropped and five hundred people sat in awe as Davis Phinney raised his arms in victory over and over on the big screen at the Victory Summit meeting in Pittsburgh during the autumn of 2012. This video introduction to our keynote speaker showed a young Davis repeatedly crossing finish lines with his hands and head held high. The deep loud voice of the narrator informed us that Davis was the winningest American cyclist of all time. The crowd was invigorated by the multiple victories of the man who won so many times that he was known as "the cash register." Even more inspiring was the speech to follow. Davis took the stage with pride. He was talking to a group of people with Parkinson's disease and their caretakers—people who understood his struggles.

Davis was just a few years older than I was when first diagnosed with Young-Onset Parkinson's disease. I couldn't imagine what it must be like for a professional athlete who depends on his body for his livelihood to lose function—or maybe I could. I too was a professional, and I too depended on my body to do my job. I braced myself for an emotional pity party—but that is not what I got.

He entered the stage and almost tripped over a speaker, jumping high in the air, and landing perfectly behind the podium. Davis smiled and said, "I did that on purpose!" He proceeded to talk about changing our mindset. Having won some major victories in his life, he said it was time to celebrate the small ones. Simple things like getting his pants on in the morning while standing were a victory. He didn't have to change my mindset. We had the same way of emotionally dealing with Parkinson's. It didn't ruin my life but changed it. It won't shorten my life—so I will live it!

Lying on my couch after my DBS surgery and watching the Beijing Olympic Games, I was impressed by a young cyclist, Taylor Phinney, who was doing well. Not a cyclist yet, I was bored by the sport, but my ears perked as the announcers mentioned that Taylor's father, Davis, had Parkinson's disease. The coverage switched to a color story on Davis who had also just been implanted with DBS. I was so inspired that I got up off the couch, went to the bike shop, and bought my first road bike.

The following summer, I got my whole family involved. The Netherlands is an incredible place for cycling. Amsterdam has more bikes than people—sixteen million over eleven million—and everybody bikes everywhere. The countryside is filled with bike trails, and well-marked and numbered destinations called *Fietspad*, which make navigation simple. Also the name Netherlands, meaning "lowlands," implied flat easy cycling. I found a bike trip with a biking tour company, and convinced the whole family to go with me.

A peloton of six families started in Amsterdam. A week later, we were in Bruges, a gorgeous city in Belgium. We pedaled at a nice, easy pace passing windmills, stopping at honey farms, and staying each night in hotels converted from ancient castles. Our picnic lunches were laid out in settings virtually painted by Monet. Wild horses and sheep escorted us through pastures. As we crossed into Belgium, the beauty of the frescoed walls along canals competed with the taste of fine chocolate.

My life was changed. My victories were new. I was living.

LEGACY

If you would not be forgotten as soon as you are dead, either write something worth reading or do things worth writing.
—Benjamin Franklin

We all spend a relatively short time in this world, and most of us would like to think that we will leave it a better place for those who follow. The same is true for me in terms of my job. I would like to think that I left the held of cardiac anesthesiology in the care of a group of young physicians who learned from my collective experience and grew from there. The truth is, we are always learning, and the held is perpetually advancing. I definitely learned as much from them as they did from me.

Over twenty years ago, as a resident, I had a mentor whose words had a great impact on me. He would always remind me that we were both doctors, just in different stages of learning. I took that to heart. I didn't need to demand respect just because I was a senior attending physician. Instead, I wanted to command respect, because I treated others with dignity and respect. I felt this way toward every member of the team, and we all worked better and learned together.

Please question me if need be. I am not the authority; the patient is most important.

This philosophy, I believe, has maximized my teaching to its full potential. I feel secure that I left behind better doctors because of our experience together, and this is reflected in letters I received from residents during that time.

Hi, Jon.

We didn't get to read your tribute during graduation, but here it is anyway. It's just a short snippet, but we want to let you know that we appreciate everything you've done for us.

Thanks for everything!

Marianne (on behalf of the 2009 Georgetown Anesthesia Class)

*****

Every now and then, a resident encounters an attending (physician) who becomes more than just a mentor. He becomes a friend. I can vouch that for every single resident in this room, both senior and junior, that attending is Jon Lessin. Jon is the kind of attending who you become Facebook friends with, the kind of attending who shares his most recent iPhone applications, the kind of attending who subscribes to satellite radio just so you can have good music in the OR, and who is not afraid to belt out lyrics to the latest Britney Spears song. Jon is, single-handedly, the reason why Georgetown residents request to go to the Washington Hospital Center, month after month. Jon is also one of the reasons why, despite three long years of indentured servitude in residency, we are all a little sad to leave.

*****

Dr. Lessin,

Congratulations on your retirement! This news saddens me for our residents, who will miss out on the opportunity to work with you, but also makes me so happy to hear that you will have more time to pursue other interests and enjoy your family after an excellent career in anesthesiology. I cant thank you enough for all of the clinical experience and knowledge you've shared. You will be greatly missed at WHC!

All the best,
Tiffany

*****

Dr. Lessin,

Thank you for the kind words, but more importantly, thank you for all the great care you have provided your patients throughout the years. Your leadership and professionalism have been a pillar of strength for the WHC Anesthesia program. We have been blessed with a tremendous opportunity to train with you and share in your passion for this great specialty. In addition to your great skills and teaching, you shared a humility and empathy that was present in each interaction with your patients. Your past trainees owe you a debt of gratitude for the role you played in our professional development. Thank you for everything, especially the respect you passed on to the residents of GUH, GW, and military programs alike. You're a first-class role model.

We wish you the best as you shift your attention to other great causes. Your energy will undoubtedly have a tremendous impact on the new lives you touch each day.

Respectfully,
Joe & Tiffany

*****

Dr. Lessin,

In case there is not a more appropriate time/ place to mention the following, I will do it here. I want to thank you for all your help last year and this year. I appreciate all of your insight and patience. I have learned so much on the cardiac rotation, and obviously love it. On a more personal note, thank you so much for the conversations we had, and for being so open about yourself and your family. You are truly an inspiration to everyone you meet, and I feel honored and privileged to know you and work with you. I have learned so much from you personally and professionally that I will carry with me throughout life. Thank you so much!

Sincerely,
Kelly

*****

Dr. Lessin,

The pleasure was ours! Listening to your wife and daughter accept the award on your behalf was the highlight of the night for many of us.

Even some of the tough guys had tears in their eyes when your daughter was at the mic! You must be proud of her. Props on the 546-mile ride, by the way. My legs hurt just thinking about it. I hope you can join us down the stretch to help present the award to future recipients.

Maggie and Adrian are next year's chief residents who will help do the selection. They are a great pair, and will see to it that the tradition continues. I envision this being a big award that anyone involved in perioperative medicine, who works closely with our residents, will be eligible for.

Thanks for everything!

*****

Jon,

I will definitely miss you at the gradua-tion dinner, but who would want to go to some stuffy grad dinner when you could be biking in the Rockies! You're getting the better end of the deal on this one for sure! Thank you for the kind e-mail. I feel so grateful to have met you, and to have had the opportunity to work with you and learn from your example as a stellar clinician and an even better human being. I have never met any-one so talented yet so humble, real, and down-to-earth. The cardiac rooms (and WHC in general) can be a hectic and stressful place where it's easy to lose your cool and lose sight of things. However, I learned a lot from your example of how to deal with situations gracefully, without losing com-posure and without taking things personally. In essence, I learned to chill out... or, rather, that I needed to chill out a bit and not get so riled up about things, but to step back and look at the big-ger picture. The younger residents have no idea what they are missing without you around.

Anyway, I wish you all the best. I'll be mov-ing to California next month, and hope to get back on my bike a bit more and explore that region.

Take care. Best regards,
Mike

*****

Thanks to all of you! I will miss you too!

AFTERWORD

Climbing to New Heights

by Jonathan Lessin, MD, and Lisa Ebb, PT, MS, NCS

All of us struggling with Parkinson's disease know that we feel better with exercise. We also know that our ability to move quickly may be dependent upon the motivation to do it. What better motivation to make a big movement, and reach quickly for a hold, than the fact that you are forty feet in the air?

I completed the LSVT BIG program two years ago, and during the intensive four-week program, I felt the best I had in ten years. I also attribute this to my DBS, medication, and hot yoga. Soon after my graduation, I realized that I was not going to do the LSVT BIG program daily without my physical therapists, Lisa and Philippe, providing the motivation. I needed to find something fun and challenging. To me, indoor rock climbing provided the same big movements, core strength, and balance as LSVT BIG, and was also challenging and rewarding. Fortunately, I found a very supportive and patient instructor, Molly, at the Sportrock Climbing Center in Alexandria.

I quickly became a rock-climbing addict. It felt good to be on the wall. While climbing, certain muscles are worked, and others stretched simultaneously. Many joints are opening and extending their range of motion. It's exhilarating! Also, there is a sense of challenge and accomplishment as you strengthen and improve your skill to ascend to harder and harder climbs in their ranking system.

We have now formed a rock-climbing group for PD, which meets on Wednesdays at 9:00 a.m., and is rapidly growing. In rock climbing, I have found the benefits of LSVT BIG therapy, and I have been able to remain motivated to do it three times weekly.

I asked my physical therapist, Lisa Ebb, how she thinks the LSVT BIG program and rock climbing could create a partnership for my continued exercise regime. She said, "The principles of the LSVT BIG program—repetitive, effortful, purposeful movement—are used with every reach and every step onto the next rock to climb to the top. Challenge and variation are the two most important principles of exercise in Parkinson's disease. I commend Jon and others who have joined him for thinking outside the box and finding challenging, vigorous activities to continue living well with Parkinson's disease."

ABOUT THE AUTHOR

An adventurer at heart, Jonathan Lessin was the cardiac anesthesiology residency director at MedStar Washington Hospital Center as well as an assistant professor of anesthesiology at Georgetown University Medical School in Washington, DC. He was the first recipient of the Lessin Award, given by the residents of the university for inspirational leadership in perioperative care.

Jonathan was diagnosed with Parkinson's at age thirty-eight, and received his deep brain stimulator at age forty-three. He became a cyclist and avid sportsman just to prove he could, despite his diagnosis.

In 2012, several years after his diagnosis, he voluntarily stepped into retirement to pursue life fulfillment. Jonathan now finds happiness encouraging his fellow "Parkies" to attempt things they thought they could never do. He currently lives in Chevy Chase with his wife and two daughters. *Tenacity* is his first published work.

CPSIA information can be obtained
at www.ICGtesting.com
Printed in the USA
FSHW02n2313270818
51626FS

9 781640 961074